Fortress NHS
A Philosophical Review of the National Health Service

David Seedhouse
University of Auckland, New Zealand
and
University of Liverpool, UK

JOHN WILEY & SONS
Chichester · New York · Brisbane · Toronto · Singapore

Copyright © 1994 by John Wiley & Sons Ltd,
Baffins Lane, Chichester,
West Sussex PO19 1UD, England
Telephone (+44) 243 779777

Other Wiley Editorial Offices

John Wiley & Sons, Inc., 605 Third Avenue,
New York, NY 10158-0012, USA

Jacaranda Wiley Ltd, 33 Park Road, Milton,
Queensland 4064, Australia

John Wiley & Sons (Canada) Ltd, 22 Worcester Road,
Rexdale, Ontario M9W 1L1, Canada

John Wiley & Sons (SEA) Pte Ltd, 37 Jalan Pemimpin #05-04,
Block B, Union Industrial Building, Singapore 2057

Library of Congress Cataloging-in-Publication Data

Seedhouse, David.
    Fortress NHS: a philosophical review of the National Health
Service / David Seedhouse.
       p.   cm.
    Includes bibliographical references and index.
    ISBN 0 471 93909 9
    1. National Health Service (Great Britain).   2. Medicine, State—Great Britain.
    3. Medical policy—Great Britain.   I. Title.
RA241.S44   1993
362.1'0941—dc20
                                                              93–30021
                                                                  CIP

British Library Cataloguing in Publication Data

A catalogue record for this book is available from the British Library

ISBN 0 471 93909 9

Typeset in 11/12pt Plantin by Vision Typesetting, Manchester
Printed and bound in Great Britain by Redwood Books, Trowbridge, Wiltshire

Contents

Preface

A war is being fought over the NHS. At first sight the battle looks straightforward – one army wants to replace state planning with a system supplying medicine through a variety of private contracts, the other is resisting any change to comprehensive health care provided equally for all. Two committed opponents, and two radical crusades – it seems that there can be only one winner, and no compromise: either the NHS will survive undamaged, or it must disintegrate.

To those fighting to defend the health service the issue is black and white. They are struggling to preserve basic principles, and the opposition is not. But the truth is not so simple. In fact both factions make regular appeal to 'the principles of the NHS', and both claim to do so sincerely. Apparently almost everyone believes that the NHS should – in some way – stand for equality, for meeting needs, for offering quality and for doing so efficiently.

The fact that fierce enemies seem to favour the same ideals is surely a phenomenon worth investigating. What do these famous principles really stand for? What intricacies of meaning are concealed by their use as slogans? And what practical implications might there be if each – once thoroughly understood – were to be applied with a view to the reform of the NHS?

Thus it is that the bulk of this book is devoted to an analysis of the ubiquitous 'NHS principles'. Perhaps surprisingly, both sides in the war will find its conclusions uncomfortable. The attackers – who would destroy the present service, and so lose many of the good things it offers – no longer have the slightest excuse for fudging matters. If they have devised a better health care system they must demonstrate the principles on which their plan is based, and explain in full why these principles trump alternatives.

However, it is the defenders who face the greatest challenge. For many years countless advocates of the British health service have taken it for granted that the 'NHS principles' are clear, sound and completely understood. So great and so sustained has this complacency been that the principles have become an unquestioned, unexamined article of faith. They have become part of a deep-seated myth which holds that the NHS is theoretically perfect and based on fundamental moral axioms. But the evidence – once properly examined – does not support the myth: not only are 'the principles' philosophically complex, and open to several different interpretations, but the NHS has never been deliberately organised in accord with them.

This book looks behind the myth, shows the complexity of the principles, and explains some of the implications of taking them seriously. Its findings must give the defenders cause to examine their faith. The defenders believe they are advocating a comprehensive health care system, but in truth they have been protecting a medical service, arranged at least partly in the interests of doctors and their suppliers. Moreover they have been defending a system which has no consistent set of purposes, and no guiding theory of health. Although many defenders believe profoundly in the 'fundamental principles', they have been fighting for a service which does not have any.

If the defenders are content with a medical NHS, and still wish to support it by the use of theory, they must explain the real principles which underpin it (for they cannot rely on the principles they thought they could). If, on the other hand, the defenders are more concerned to maintain *the principles demonstrated in this book* – and wish to create an NHS truly in keeping with these principles – they must change their colours and argue against the NHS as it is today.

This is not to say that a national medical service is undesirable. On the contrary, properly organised medical care can be an important factor in the drive to work for health: but it is not the only factor, nor is it necessarily always primary. What is more, the way the NHS is organised at present – as a fortress defending itself against all comers, hoping to grab as much of the national welfare budget as possible – means that *rational planning in health care is a practical impossibility*.

The defenders do not have to choose whether or not to join the attackers in their quest for private medicine. But they do have to decide if they want to rebel against their own assumptions and certainties. If they accept that they have been trying to preserve a medical system which they thought had principles but which they now realise does not, they must change their position. Converts to the idea of a health service truly working for health must argue for full-scale reform. They can continue to be against further tinkering with a nationalised medical system, but what really matters is that they come to be *for* massive change in the theory and practice of public health care. Those who wish to campaign for a rational and philosophically justifiable national health service must now determine where they stand. Are they happy to argue only that a government-owned medical service should continue much as it has in the past – or would they rather work for the creation of the first real health service in Britain?

A note to the reader. The trend in almost all literature about the NHS is to regard expressions such as 'medical services' and 'health services', 'medical need', 'health need' and 'health care need' as always interchangeable. In fact they are not. However, to avoid over-use of quotation marks, this fallacy is not *always* challenged in this book.

Acknowledgements

During the time in which this book was being planned and written I was supported by many kind people in ways which most of them will scarcely remember. I do though, and I thank them. Of those who have helped directly with the development of my ideas I am especially grateful to Ian Buchanan, who introduced me to the distinction between process and purpose in the health service, and to my Masters students who enrolled at Liverpool University in 1990. This unforgettably pleasant and tolerant group helped immensely with the initial clarification of my ideas, and enabled me to continue at those times when it might have been easier to give up.

In addition, I would like to thank my publisher, and particularly my editor, Verity Waite, for their constancy and friendly encouragement with this, and other projects. I am also grateful to the University of Auckland, for whom I was employed during the later stages of this work. The University made the transition from life in my home country to life in a foreign land far smoother, and so more productive, than I could possibly have imagined. Above all I am grateful to Hilary for her immense support.

On looking back at books, once the dust has settled, key events which occurred during their writing invariably spring to mind. Undoubtedly, when I come to pick up *Fortress NHS* in future years I shall remember the University of Central Lilliput and its induction programme into the Twilight Zone of HE. I might also recall a chance remark overheard in a corridor that from time to time one encounters places which are to academia what Captain Scarlet is to undertaking. Experiences do not always have to be enjoyable to be formative.

Part One: A Purposeful Organisation?

Dialogue One

The Managers' Problem

*It has just turned nine o'clock. Six men in sharp suits, and two powerfully dressed women, are sitting in a recently refurbished board room. A black oak table dents a deep carpet while vertical blinds slice the winter sun. The group is working through a packed agenda, and has reached **Item 5: Budgetary re-allocation within the Hospital**. Dr Graham, the director of the Hospital Trust, is 'talking to' a previously circulated discussion paper – a proposal to close the long-stay geriatric ward.*

Dr Graham: . . . so I think you are bound to agree that the figures speak for themselves . . . (*He half raises a hand from the table, in a general gesture*) . . . if I may I'll take questions after my summary.

In essence my case has four main planks: first, nursing the elderly in hospital incurs excessive labour costs; second, almost all patients could be moved either to local authority nursing homes, or better still to their own homes where family care is the preferred option; third, with Jones due to retire in 18 months we could create a consultant post in an extra-contractual referral trigger specialism (ERTS); and fourth, there's minimum danger of fuss or outcry. There's not a lot of media mileage in geriatrics, and nowadays everybody accepts that resources are limited. When there's not enough to go around tough decisions have to be made. Nobody likes doing it, but these days everyone sees the need for it. Comments anyone?

Melanie Smith (*the most junior member of the management team*)*:* Well, I agree that it is certainly a possibility, but I don't think we should necessarily see it as the best choice straightaway. There has been a fair amount of controversy about the quality of care in the community recently, and there's a growing lobby arguing that institutions are actually safer and happier places for many old people. Also, I wonder if it might not appear to some that we always impose cuts on the softest option. I can't remember the last time we looked really seriously at the budget for surgery, but here we are talking about an entire ward closure . . . (*she hesitates*).

Dr Graham: Go on.

Melanie Smith: I hope you don't mind but Donald and I (*she nods towards her colleague*) were so interested in your discussion paper that we called a Quality Task Force (QTF) meeting. We explored some of the issues and came up with two key proposals. One was that we'd like to adjourn Item 5 for two weeks to allow time for Quality Department Groups (QDGs) to design a needs-assessment programme . . .

Dr Graham: No, we must decide swiftly. What was your other idea?

Melanie Smith: The other was that we invite the hospital ethicist to explore this agenda item with us today.

Donald Arthur: (*quickly*) We appreciate that this is rather an unusual step, but since this is clearly an ethical issue, and none of us has qualifications in ethics, we thought he might have some useful pointers for us.

Dr Graham: I didn't know we had an ethicist. When was he appointed?

Donald Arthur: Only fairly recently in fact, in line with central directives. But he has been fully briefed, and he realises that we can only see him for a short time.

Dr Graham: I doubt that it will do any good. But if you insist? Very well, 15 minutes maximum.

The ethicist, who has been waiting outside, is called into the meeting.

Ethicist: Good morning. How can I help you?

Dr Graham: (*in avuncular fashion*) I'm not sure you can, but Melanie here seems to think we have an ethical problem on our hands.

Ethicist: Naturally you do. Within the present NHS set up, there will inevitably be many ethical problems.

Dr Graham: No doubt you are right, but we'd prefer it if you would concentrate your advice on the problem in hand. We want to hear your views on whether or not it is ethical to shut the ward.

Ethicist: I can't possibly answer that question directly. There are so many other factors which must be taken into account. If the problem is to be properly understood it is essential that you analyse these factors. My job, as I see it, is to facilitate your analysis by posing clear and demanding questions.

Peter Walker: Excuse me, but you are not here to ask questions, and I'm sure we all think perfectly clearly already. You are here, as a specialist ethicist, to give us answers. What's the most ethical solution to our dilemma?

Ethicist: If you don't mind I'd rather you didn't call me an 'ethicist'. As you cast it the problem before us appears to be a standard ethical dilemma (of the 'where should the axe fall next?' variety) but it is in fact a much deeper problem. In order to demonstrate its essential nature it must be explored philosophically. You seem to want your 'ethicist' to give you a simple answer to a simple problem. But yours is not a simple problem. It is highly complex, and until the extent of this complexity has been uncovered there is no hope of getting an adequate solution.

Dr Graham: Nonsense. We have simple solutions open to us. We can shut the ward, we can make cost-improvements elsewhere instead, we can charge the patients for 'hotel services', or we can reduce staffing levels across the hospital. These are simple solutions. All you have to do is tell us, in your opinion, which of these is the most ethically defensible.

Philosopher: Those are simplistic solutions. They don't really solve anything. They just push the problem off somewhere else. You will not get truly valuable solutions until you understand the context of the problem, just as a chess player can never intentionally come up with an interesting and original strategy unless she thoroughly understands the nature of the game she is playing. The best thing I can do is to help you understand the context of your work better. Why, for instance, are any of you here at all?

Dr Graham: I presume you mean why are we gathered around this particular table, and what our work responsibilities are – not anything more existential. The meaning of life would be a little heavy for a Monday morning.

Philosopher: Is there a bad time to discuss the subject? Why is it inappropriate for health service employees to talk about the meaning of life? What could be more natural?

Dr Graham: We are here to make a hard decision, not to engage in abstract discussion.

Philosopher: But you are about to make a huge decision about the lives of a great many people. Surely one of the factors that you must consider is what life means for each of these people. I see that as very concrete.

Dr Graham: We cannot go into that sort of detail.

Philosopher: Detail? The meaning of life is a detail?

Dr Graham: No. What I mean is that our decision is at the macro-level. We are concerned with the hospital budget. We are concerned to allocate resources effectively according to clinical, managerial and economic criteria. We cannot go into the intricacies of the life of each individual.

Philosopher: There you go again. The meaning of life is now an intricacy.

Dr Graham: It's an intricate question.

Philosopher: I agree, but what you really meant was that there are big questions with which you are concerned around this table and a subsidiary question which is the meaning of life.

Dr Graham: We are none of us here to play games.

Philosopher: Perhaps we should return to my question then. Let me put it to you in a slightly different fashion: for what main purpose, or purposes, are you employed within this hospital? Dr Graham, would you like to start?

Dr Graham: Certainly. I think we should all lay our cards face up on the table. I'm here because I get paid very well to be here. I've worked hard to get where I am, I like the job, I have power, I have responsibilities, I enjoy making decisions.

Philosopher: Thank you for your honesty. I think those are important – and common – impulses, but they are not the only ones surely?

Melanie Smith: No they are not. We are trying to do a difficult job in the best interests of the patients, in fact in the best interests of the whole community who might make use of our hospital. The basic reason we are here is to promote health, and to do so fairly.

Simon Guthrie: Yes, and it is not easy. It means we have to make painful decisions. Perhaps it would be better to say that we do our best to be fair.

Dr Graham: Quite. And Simon might have gone on to say that the hospital is not here solely for the patients either. A lot of good people work here. I myself spend most of my waking life in the place. The staff have interests and priorities too – let's not forget that – we undertake clinical research, our doctors add to the fund of medical knowledge, and we also educate medical students within these walls.

Philosopher: Thank you. That's a lot of purposes already: health, the interests of the patients, medical education, fairness, justice, improving knowledge, and self-interest.

I suppose you might add monitoring and surveillance of population trends, health education, disease prevention work, reducing costs wherever possible, giving clear explanations to patients, and a host of others we would come up with if we thought for a while longer. There are so many purposes here that I think we need to distinguish between the more or less important, if we can. Or do you think all these purposes are equally important?

Melanie Smith: I wouldn't care to judge between them.

Philosopher: But you don't mind judging about whether or not to close a ward?

Donald Arthur: That's not fair. It's because of Melanie that you were asked here at all. She wants to make sure that the geriatric patients get a fair deal.

Melanie Smith: Yes. If I have to judge then I will put the patient first.

Philosopher: Rhetoric.

Melanie Smith: What?

Philosopher: It seems to be a rule of life in the health service that as soon as a conversation begins to touch on anything difficult or philosophical everyone leaps for cover in rhetoric. 'We're all working for patient well-being' or 'We're against inequalities in health' or 'We must save the health service' or 'We all have a right to health'. If anyone then asks you what you mean some sort of intelligent answer is the least that might be expected. Instead, what happens? Anyone who dares to be curious, anyone who has the courage to stand outside the waffle is either ignored, ridiculed or stamped on for rocking the boat. Anything rather than answer his question.

Melanie, the whole reason you asked me here is that it is not possible always to 'put the patient first' if this means always doing the very best for each patient. This is your whole problem so it's hardly an answer to ignore it.

Melanie Smith: I'm big enough to take that. There is a lot of rhetoric spoken in discussions about the health service. Some of us are aware of that. We're looking to you to help us begin to debate in a more substantial way. Because we resort to what you call rhetoric it doesn't mean that we want to hide behind it. Most of us have not been trained to think philosophically. Some of us are brave enough to admit it. It's very scary to confess that you don't know the answer. You might at least give me some credit for this.

Philosopher: I am sorry. Sometimes I let exasperation get the better of me too easily. What I'm trying to get at is that no manager in the health service faced with a resource allocation problem can have it both ways. It is inconsistent to say that all purposes are equal and at the same time use ranked criteria, albeit implicitly, to make crucial resource allocation decisions.

Dr Graham: I see. In other words you are saying that if we discuss our purposes openly, and decide which are the most important, then we will have a better understanding of how we should allocate resources?

Philosopher: Yes.

Dr Graham: Good. Then what we need to do now is to list our purposes in order of preference and then we'll be on our way to some guidelines. We might even come up with a Code of Practice. I see what you are getting at now.

Philosopher: I don't think it will be as easy as that. If you are serious about letting me give you some guidance then we have a major project on our hands. It's not something we can undertake in a single meeting. In fact it may not be possible ever to reach a satisfactory ending to it.

Dr Graham: We don't have the time for any more meetings. That is a fact of life.

Donald Arthur: I'm sorry but I think the problem deserves more time. We do need help with decisions like this, and we seem to be facing them more and more often these days.

Dr Graham: Very well, since some of you are expressing an unusual level of interest in this issue I suggest you get together to form a working party, with the ethicist, but you must report to me by the end of this week. Is this acceptable to you?

Philosopher: Yes, I shall do my best. But before you move on can I ask, if there is to be a working group, could the members consider a briefing paper? I think I could adapt some earlier work and circulate it by this afternoon . . .

Paper One

Purpose

In order to ensure that consistent decisions are made in the National Health Service it is essential for all policy-makers to have a clear view of the purpose, or purposes, of the organisation. At the moment no such view exists. But without one, while some specific local policies may be clear and firm, NHS planning overall must continue to be vague. If this situation is to be improved, as it must be if NHS resources are to be used most effectively, it is vital to understand its causes.

Moving Targets

The NHS contains an enormous range of interest groups. Sometimes these groups have shared goals, but not always. At one time or another every party comes into competition with others. For example, NHS managers are charged with the task of keeping service costs to a minimum while clinicians feel duty bound to fight for increases in their individual budgets. Furthermore, since resources are limited the professional goals of one set of doctors are bound, sooner or later, to conflict with those of colleagues.[1] Outside the medical realm many nurses seek to advocate on behalf of patients but are often prevented from doing so by tight staffing levels and – not uncommonly – by resistance from others with different priorities.[2,3] Patients too, often have their objectives confounded. In illness many people wish for tranquillity, time to talk, and the space and opportunity in which to learn as much as possible about what is happening to them, but for many reasons these needs cannot always be met.[4]

The list of practical conflicts of purpose in the health service is potentially endless. By itself this is not a problem, nor is it unusual. Clashes of interest are inevitable within any complex organisation. Similar political struggles occur daily in supermarket chains, banks and factories but in the case of the NHS there is one quite fundamental difference. The essential purpose of business activity is known and agreed, but in the health service it is not. In business, financial profit is the ultimate measure of success and is easily calculated, but the profit of health work is far more difficult to evaluate. Businesses have accountants to tell them how successful they are, but while there are nowadays many accountants working in the health service there are no accountants of health care.

If the NHS were the equivalent of a commercial enterprise then it would be possible to place it in the same category as a supermarket chain. But this comparison cannot withstand serious scrutiny, as this reported conversation between a health service manager and the managing director of Sainsbury shows:

> I went to see Roy Griffiths in his office at Sainsbury's (sic) and while I was talking to him, his secretary handed him a piece of paper. He looked at it and said, 'OK'. I asked him, 'What do you mean "OK"?' and he said, 'My organisation is OK today'. It turned out he had just six measures on that piece of paper and from those he could tell what the state of Sainsbury's health had been the day before; things like the amount of money taken yesterday, the freshness quotient – the amount of stuff still on the shelves, the proportion of staff on duty, and so on.[5]

Naturally, an efficient industry such as Sainsbury ought to be able to distil its measures of success or failure into simple types. And at first glance it does not seem unreasonable to assume that the same thing should be possible with the NHS. Conventional wisdom has it that this is not possible at the moment simply because there are just not enough data available.[6] Employ sufficient people to dig up enough facts and figures, expose all the costs and benefits to scrutiny and the managing director of the NHS will also be able to say 'my organisation is OK today' on reading a few measures on a piece of A4. But this is a pipe-dream. Even if every possible item of 'health service outcome' could be recorded, health service planners would be no closer to the position of the supermarket manager. Indeed, the more information they obtain about the many benefits which health work can help produce, the further away they become from the commercial ideal.

In contrast to the retail world, in health care it is as if there is a range of possible goals and targets, suspended in solution. From time to time, from place to place, and for one reason or another, these targets move up or down in the solution – none is at the bottom all the time and none is permanently at the top. What is more the solution can be shaken up by the turn of events – for instance, it can be disturbed by the application of economic measures such as the Quality Adjusted Life Year (QALY), or by the installation of management. Numerous influences – ranging from the power of clinicians to external commercial pressure – can act to move the targets higher or lower, in accord with how important each perceives them to be. There is no fixed pattern, and apparently no overriding objective reason to have the targets in one position rather than another. Thus, while it is quite feasible for managers in business to work to improve the success of their organisations (since they already know the general hierarchy of their targets), life is quite different for NHS planners, who lack certainty about even the most primitive question, 'what are we in operation for?'.

No Clear Theory of Health – No Consensus on Purpose

A large part of the disorientation of the NHS can be explained by the fact that the meaning of health continues to be opaque and disputed. Countless books and articles have explored this central issue, yet it is consistently ignored by most policy-makers in the NHS.[7] The basic problem is that while most theories of health contend that health is 'more than the absence of disease' and that health work is consequently more than medical work, the health service is dominated by medical interests and priorities. This picture is further complicated by the fact that while some medical workers prefer to concentrate on the science of medicine, many others believe that health work transcends clinical activity and consequently seek – as a legitimate part of their professional role – to communicate well, to consider people's lives in social context, and sometimes even aim to befriend their patients.[8] Thus some doctors set the limits of their health work in one place while others draw the line quite differently, and so not all doctors have the same priorities either in theory or practice.

Such variations in opinion are not restricted to the medical profession. Other health workers too disagree about which theory of health should govern their activities: as a general rule the less technical the discipline the broader the notion of health espoused. Some theories of health focus on morbidity and mortality but others[9] espouse well-being, empowerment, and even happiness. However, these different ideas cannot be combined in every circumstance. Disease cure cannot always be had at the same time as well-being,[10] greater fitness does not lead to greater control in all circumstances,[11] and sometimes longer life just means extended misery. Whatever theoretical criterion of health (or purpose) is selected by one group of people there will, quite commonly, be good reasons for others to dispute it. Consequently, while different groups may each claim to be working for health, in reality their purposes can be quite different.

Muddy History, Muddled Principles

In order to understand how the NHS is able to operate without a consistent hierarchy of purpose it is essential to know a little of its history. Contrary to what many Britons have come to believe:

> The National Health Service did not spring, like Athene fully armed, from the head of Aneurin Bevan but was a point of rapid change in continuing growth.[12]

Indeed, according to several historians the NHS was hardly designed at all. There never was a clear blueprint for the organisation, and its practical structure immediately after enactment was much the same as before. The essential difference was ambition:

> The National Health Service Act is best seen as an indication of the sort of service then thought desirable, rather than as a description of provisions which were actually being made.[13]

The story of the Act began before the start of World War II. As early as 1938 a small group of civil servants were already considering the future development of national health services. At this time help in sickness was not guaranteed and the chance of receiving treatment varied according to the nature of the disease, extent of insurance cover, and the place of residence of the sick person. In Bevan's words:

> . . . our hospital organisation has grown up with no plan, with no system; it is unevenly distributed over the country and indeed it is one of the tragedies of the situation that very often the best hospital facilities are available where they are least needed. In the older industrial districts of Great Britain hospital facilities are inadequate. Many of the hospitals are too small – very much too small.[14]

By 1939 it was widely agreed that this situation was neither efficient nor equitable, and that what was required instead was a planned health care system to make 'the best means of maintaining health and curing disease' available 'to all citizens'.[15] The only question was how this might best be achieved. But on this there was no consensus.[16] In principle, two quite different strategies for achieving change were possible:

> One, with all the attraction of simplicity, would be to disregard the past and the present entirely and to invent *ad hoc* a completely new reorganisation for all health requirements. The other is to use and absorb the experience of the past and the present, building it into a wider service.[17]

However, despite the appeal of rebuilding post-war society with a clean sheet, conservative thinking was dominant. Thus, three developments based on existing systems were considered. The first was to extend the existing National Health Insurance scheme to further sections of the community. This would, given the purchase of appropriate insurance entitlements, ensure the right of individuals to medical care through general practitioners. The second was to develop local authority services (whose areas of responsibility already included medical treatment within municipal hospitals, chronic care for the elderly, institutions for the mentally ill, maternity clinics, and the health of schoolchildren) so as to guarantee better public health for the community as a whole. But it was the third option which prevailed. This was:

> . . . the suggestion that the hospitals of England and Wales should be administered as a National Health Service by the Ministry.[18]

A Missed Chance

If the opportunity to define health properly had been taken in the 1940s, and a new national health service had been designed from a philosophically clear base, a more intelligible institution might have emerged. But the chance was lost. Despite the fact that the 1944 White Paper and 1946 Act in places seem to favour a broad notion of health the idea was never given substance, and the NHS turned out to be little more than a medical service dressed up in fine language. According to Rudolf Klein, an authority on social policy:

> . . . the 1948 NHS was essentially a hospital service . . .[19]

> . . . designed to accommodate certain specific interests within the medical profession . . . (who) . . . obtained a monopoly of legitimacy among the health service providers: a unique position, reflected in the participation of doctors in the running of the NHS.[20]

Thus the NHS began as a non-philosophical fudge and has persisted in like fashion for nearly five decades. But by building on a philosophically muddled past, where health care had come to be synonymous with medical services,[21] the architects of the NHS were guaranteeing an equally mixed up, medically governed future.

Tensions Within

For a while the political fudge concealed a number of tensions. However, while the creation of the NHS enabled all interested parties to feel some satisfaction at the time, their goals may ultimately be impossible to harmonise. For Klein the 1948 NHS embodied not only a clash of professional interests, but also a clash of values. He maintains that the values of 'rationality, efficiency and equity' won out in 1948, but also sees that there was then, and is now, another set of values within the service. Klein describes them as:

> . . . responsiveness rather than efficiency, differentiation rather than uniformity, self-government rather than national equity . . .[20]

He believes that the two sets of beliefs, and the different policies they tend to inspire, could be fundamentally contradictory:

> Some of these contradictions reflected political concessions: the deliberate acceptance of imperfections in the grand design in order to minimise opposition. Other contradictions, however, reflected the incompatibility of certain objectives. The history of the NHS since 1948 can largely be seen as the working out of these contradictions: a continuing and never-ending attempt to reconcile what may well turn out to be irreconcilable aims of policy.[20]

No doubt Klein is right that there are two very different organisational ideologies at work in the NHS, and that these are based in radically different political outlooks: the one favouring central planning and the other regional freedom of action. But the contradiction and incompatibility of objectives is even greater than it appears from his perspective. It is not just that there are competing political schools debating how best to achieve the same general end – all want to deliver the best health care but cannot agree on the means. The essential problem is that the end itself is seen quite differently by the many different groups which operate within the British health care system.

Political Compromise and Philosophical Complacency

In order to satisfy the disparate goals of various interested parties it is often considered politically undesirable to state one's purpose specifically. In this rather cynical light the memorable phrases in the official documents of the 1940s may seem to have at least as much to do with compromise and appeasement as with exact policy.* It is not difficult to concur in principle with

---

* Such an interpretation would seem difficult to sustain in full. While it is true that the formative documents were not specific, they do have a far-sightedness quite lacking in their more modern counterparts.

the aspiration to a service which '. . . is available to all people and . . . covers all necessary forms of health care . . .'[17] because the phrase can be understood in many different ways. Precisely what must be available to everyone?

What forms of health care are necessary and which not? Answers to these questions cannot be found in government writings of the time, and they certainly are not in evidence today.

However, even though the conceptual foundations of the NHS are demonstrably obscure the British people have, over the last half century, indulged in a massive act of collective delusion and complacency. For all this time virtually everyone has taken it for granted that the hard philosophical work has been done – the basic governing principles precisely laid out and appropriate practical policies derived. This act of blind faith has been so great and so sustained that even in 1991 it was possible to write, apparently with absolute conviction:

> Show your belief in an NHS that is Fair: Equal: Caring: Comprehensive.[22]

But these ideas have never been thought through in sufficient depth or with enough clarity to be applicable. What is a fair health service? How comprehensive is 'comprehensive'? In what sense should a health service be equal? The problem is not only that answering these questions is immensely difficult, but also that there are many alternative, plausible answers possible. Until the range of possibilities is fully explored, and until the options have been thoroughly analysed, the direction of the NHS must remain in doubt.

The Four NHS Principles

Very many people have written and said a great deal against what they imagine to be attacks on the 'basic principles' of the NHS, but no-one appears to be able to say with any precision what these principles are. However, with a little philosophical licence it is possible to outline the popular essence of the 'central principles', and to trace the themes back to the idealism of the 1940s.

The 1944 White Paper said:

> The proposed service must be 'comprehensive' in two senses – first that it is available to all people and, second, that it covers all necessary forms of health care'.

In addition, elsewhere in the formative official papers – as well as in later government documents – it is possible to find several statements to the effect that the 'best services' should be provided.[17,23,24]

This collection of sentiments, in one form or another, has come to be common currency amongst NHS commentators, whether they support or are opposed to the service. The basic set of NHS principles continues to emphasise 'meeting needs', 'equality' and 'access to the best services', and now contains one additional principle. At the formation of the NHS it was expected that, as the expanded service dealt with a reservoir of 'unmet need', demand for health services would steadily fall off. But of course this did not happen and demand for medical services has grown constantly ever since, and appears insatiable.[25,26]

This hunger for health services is now taken as a fact of life, and has led to the virtually universal consensus in the developed world that health service spending must be kept in check. Hence the fourth principle: that in pursuit of the other three the costs of health care should be contained.

The Conventional Set

Given the persisting vagueness which surrounds the principles it is unlikely that everyone will agree that the four phrases below do, in fact, accurately describe the conventional set. However, these or reasonably similar statements seem to occur more than any others in the voluminous literature on the NHS. Thus, the four principles of the NHS can be taken to be:

---

1. The NHS should meet all health needs

2. Everyone should receive the best care

3. The NHS should be egalitarian

4. The costs of health care should be kept as low

   as possible

Fig. 1

Conflicting Principles

To many the aim to meet all health needs, equally, with quality, and at as little cost to the national purse as possible is an admirable ambition. However, even spelt out in the above very general fashion the principles do not hold together, and cannot always all be had at once. More often than not, in practice working to achieve one of them entails working against another. Sustained philosophical analysis is necessary to gain a proper understanding of the depth of the four principles, but their basic incompatibility can nevertheless be demonstrated at a simple level.

These are some of the most obvious tensions:

1. When sought in tandem goals two and four (to offer the best care at lowest cost) are extremely difficult to reconcile. If, as a matter of principle, everyone should receive care of the highest quality, and if most functions of the NHS cost money in one way or another (which is clearly true), and if best care is

more expensive than care of a lower quality (as is usually the case), then financial costs cannot be kept to a minimum. It is simply not possible to seek the best of care and strive for serious cost-containment at the same time, without either distorting or compromising the notion of 'best care' or 'quality', or spending more than the minimum.

2. Goals one and three (that all health needs should be met and that everyone should have equal access to health services – which is one interpretation of egalitarianism) can be had only in a hypothetical world where there are unlimited resources, or where the 'set of health needs' is small and clearly delimited. In reality only some sorts of health needs are met by the NHS,[27,28] and some people receive health services before others – for instance, some people are able to pay for private medicine, some may be more familiar with the system than others, or some may be judged more suitable by those in charge of admission – to give but a few 'discriminating factors'.

The following is illuminating:

'Among the factors that influence the allocation of hospital resources in Britain, . . . (are) . . . the following:
1. *age* – for example, lack of routine access of the elderly to chronic dialysis;
2. *fear of the disease* – radiotherapy for cancer is readily available;
3. *visibility* – hemophilia, which is visible, is more widely treated than angina pectoris, which is not;
4. *aggregate costs* – hemophilia is expensive but there are only a few new cases each year;
5. *capital funds cost* – CT scanners are scarce because of large acquisition and maintenance costs;
6. *costs of alternatives* – hip replacements are done because the alternative care of a disabled patient is higher than the costs of the procedure'.[29]

Where resources are scarce (for whatever reason) it is not possible either to guarantee everyone an 'equal service' or to offer an assurance that all health needs will be met, even when people are in 'equal need'. Decisions have to be made about which services to provide, and which groups to target. The reality is that some people in certain circumstances (for example, those who qualify for mammographies and those living in well-served localities) will get better services than others.

Even in theory goals one and three are not attainable since what does and does not count as a 'health need' is not clear. Nor is it obvious that people with an identical clinical problem (which is held by some to be a necessary condition for the existence of health need) should be treated equally. For example, one of two people with an identical medical condition may – for some reason – be better placed to cope with it.

3. Recently in the UK 'freedom of choice' has been mooted as a means to control costs in the NHS. It has been suggested that this notion can justify both 'internal competition' between 'purchasers and providers', and legislation to enable patients to contract freely with doctors and other health workers. Part of the thinking is that competition will keep prices down, and also that the freedom to choose is desirable in principle.

However, under this philosophy goals three and four are not compatible. Under market rules, just as people with higher paid jobs can buy bigger cars and better houses if they wish, so patients (and other purchasers) with greater resources can contract for better health services than their poorer neighbours. Financial costs may be kept down through such freedom of choice, but at the cost of equal access. On the other hand, if controls are built in to ensure equal distribution where resources are limited, then free choice is bound to be considerably curtailed since the range of options will have to be reduced for the sake of ensuring equality of provision of 'the core'. Essentially 'equality' and a truly free market in health services are simply incompatible notions – one requires planning and control of what is available and who can have it first, while the other simply allows the size of personal wealth, and what people choose to do with that wealth, to dictate what health services can be had.

The tremendously complicated and blatantly inequitable system in the US bears perfect testimony to this incompatibility.[30]

The relationship between these principles is considerably more complicated than this preliminary survey shows. More extensive analysis reveals many more conceptual difficulties but, happily, can also show the way to a more coherent system.

Dialogue Two

Different Tribes?

It is now Tuesday. Five managers and the philosopher are seated comfortably around a low table which holds a steaming decanter of freshly percolated coffee. Outside a chill wind intermittently hurls a clatter of rain at the angular windows. The philosopher, who is facing the windows, can see the faded orange curtains of the obstetric ward in the opposite tower, and when he leans forward can just catch sight of the top of the skyscraper through the heavy drizzle.

Melanie Smith: Can I ask if everybody has had the opportunity to read the briefing paper? Good. Does anyone wish to raise any points at this stage, or shall I simply ask the author to explain how his thinking can help us with our problem?

Peter Walker: Yes, I'd like to say something. I'm worried about two points. First of all I can't see how this abstract thinking about health service purpose and principles has any useful bearing on our problem. We have to make a decision by Friday about our geriatric ward. A potted history of the health service, and the philosopher demonstrating that **he** is confused about our fundamental principles, seems a very long way from our dilemma. Our principles are very clear. They only become hard to understand if people try to be too clever. Secondly, reading the paper made me question whether the philosopher has a role with us at all. I think we must agree that there is some point to our mini-series of meetings or call it a day right now.

Philosopher: I'm sorry but I thought the paper explained perfectly clearly how, in order to make sensible policy decisions, it is necessary to clarify the basic theory and direction of health care. Unless this is done first any policy decision will be arbitrary to some degree. Think about your colleagues in the hospitals across the county. You know better than I do that if they come to be faced with a similar problem to you they might very well reach a quite different decision, and the essential reason for this is not practical differences – although there are bound to be some – but the lack of a general theory to which everyone can turn for guidance.

Peter Walker: I realise that's more or less what you wrote, but I don't think you proved your point. Policy decisions are taken all the time in the health service, and they are not **that** different in different areas. I think the basic problem is not lack of theory but lack of money. If the government gave us more money we would not be considering any ward closures.

Philosopher: I don't think financial restrictions are your main problem, although of course they make it very difficult to run a hospital, especially when that hospital contains so many interests and motivations. However much money you have someone would surely think of a way to spend it, and just as surely someone else would object. The more money put into the NHS the more tests, the more experiments, the more research of doubtful value, the more commercial pressure to invest in new drugs and machinery there will be. What you need is a way to make sense of the health service, a way to think about goals and allocate resources rationally rather than in an inconsistent fashion. . . .

Simon Guthrie: Forgive me for interrupting but I think there is a fundamental issue which you fail to see. Let me say first that I did enjoy your paper, and there's clearly something in what you say – certainly the history of the NHS is a lot more murky than most people think. No, it's the philosophical stuff which bothers me. The way you think, and the way you seem to be suggesting that we address our problem just doesn't fit with the way we do things in the NHS. Let me put it this way. I think Peter is right. It may be that, through no fault of your own or of your discipline, you can be of no help to us because we do not really think in the same ways. You are obviously a clear thinking person, but the fact is that we do not do clear thinking around here. I admit it – we fudge and we compromise, sooner or later we cloud everything. And the reason we do this is to survive in a difficult, far from perfect world.

So what you are trying to do with us is a hopeless task. We just are not capable of dissecting ourselves as I think you want us to, but we can nevertheless do useful work. When we run up against certain kinds of problem, then you might be able to help us. Perhaps it **is** only the ethical problems where you have a role. Here you can help us think through our problems and arrive at the most acceptable solutions, for instance you might be able to convince us that the old people will be much more seriously harmed than we think if we close the ward. If so this will be a valuable contribution, but any more than this is beyond your scope.

Philosopher (slowly): What you are saying is that for the most part what you do and what I do are incommensurable . . . This is a very important point, and I'm not at all sure that you are not right. It might turn out that I can be of no help to you, but I would like to try nevertheless. I think that at the very least there must be points of contact between us – we are communicating at the moment after all. Perhaps I should spell out where I think the problem lies, so that we can be as clear as possible about where we stand.

You, all of you, are here now not because you particularly want to be but because you have been told to be here. You are all very busy and have a lot of different, difficult decisions to make today – never mind worry for too long about the major judgement you will have to make collectively on Friday. You know that the reality of the health service is bargaining, politics, keeping the right people happy, acting on briefs and policies that you don't necessarily agree with, using language that you would be embarrassed to use in front of your non-NHS friends – basically you accept that you must toe the line and be inconsistent in order to survive – this is what the culture of the health service is.

After people have been immersed in any culture for a while they begin to adopt its ways and patterns of thinking and behaviour as if these are generally normal. As such you are not too different from any other tribe, and if studied by sociologists and anthropologists **as a tribe** you would throw up the same general results as any other 'sub-culture'. You have your systems, you have your beliefs – they may not make much sense to people from other systems but they make sense to you and that's what matters.

Of course I too have been trained in a highly esoteric fashion. I have been taught that all systems of belief which do not use reason and logic in the way my system does are inferior. They are mistaken to the extent to which they are inconsistent, muddled, confused, and unable to justify their activities and processes. From my perspective I find your system very mistaken indeed – it has clearly developed out of political expedience rather than according to a reasoned plan. The way I propose to tackle your problem then is not, and cannot be, to join your system, but to show you how you seem to be confused from where I stand, and to help dismantle your 'unreason'. This way you might have real and lasting ways to solve your problems. I will not go so far as to say that through my method you will find the one right way to direct your energies, but I should at least be able to show you a coherent framework for development. If I am successful I will be able to suggest a solid rather than transient answer to your current dilemma. Don't you think this is worth a try?

Simon Guthrie: I'm not convinced, you could just be wrong you know. For instance, you say that the NHS isn't a business but it very obviously is a business in many respects. Every time you consult your GP you go to a businessman, as you must know since you've read up on health service history.

Philosopher: Yes, of course I accept that many people in the NHS see what they do as business activity, but not everyone sees health work like this. And this wasn't my main point. The basic conceptual problem is to do with the differences in the general sets of purposes of straightforward commercial companies, and the NHS. Where an ordinary business – let's say it's a football club – has a broadly coherent set of purposes, the NHS does not. Of course a football club contains divergent interests, but it is not difficult to have a general understanding of the purpose of the club. Success, for a football club, rests on winning competitions, and playing in a way which will attract customers through the turnstiles. If this can be achieved then further success is either more of the same, or expansion in some other way. If this cannot be achieved then it is enough to remain in business and to hope for greater future success, during which time it is enough to provide work for the employees and interest for those spectators who stay loyal.

Each member of the football club might be thought of as having a 'defined field' of rationality, which will contain such goals as personal success, team success, higher wages, constant selection to the first team and so on. Within this 'defined field' there may be many goals, not all of which can be had together, but which the member will organise so as to ensure the more general goal, or at least not endanger it.

Perhaps the easiest way to think of the idea of a 'defined field' is to imagine a person on a boat, working together with a fleet of other boats. This person will have all sorts of goals – relaxing, competing, cooking, reading, navigating, communicating with others and so on – not all of which he can achieve at once, so he will work out ways to organise his many rational goals. The fleet, including the smaller boat, might be thought of as moving towards a shared general goal – with the lesser activities in all the boats each contributing, in some way, towards this movement.

I think such a picture applies to commercial enterprises in general. However, in the NHS while it is correct to think of each rational person as having a range of commensurable activities within her 'defined field', all of which will be contributing to her general set of work goals, the boats of individuals in the NHS fleet are not like the boats of football club members. Without wishing to sound too corny, they are not all directed towards the same harbour (even though each wants to stay afloat, and each sees the sense of staying in the main fleet). A successful footballer will usually belong to a successful club, but a successful nurse need not belong to a successful hospital – it may be that the achievement of her basic aims (perhaps one of her central goals will be to develop a ward on which research is undertaken primarily for the sake of status) will contradict the success of the hospital – if such a phrase has any meaning. Of course, the same may apply to the footballer who enjoys personal fame and fortune while his club dwindles. But in the case of the footballer it will quite soon be clear that his boat is moving in a different direction to that of the football club as a whole. If collective success is to be had then either the footballer must change his ways, or must be sold. One major difference is that although this will be obvious at the club it will not be at the hospital since what counts as overall success will not be clear (you might say the fleet will be sailing on, but will not know which harbour, or even coastline, to aim for).

Peter Walker: What are you talking about?

Philosopher: I'm trying to explain that what has to be done to solve your practical problem is first for everyone to be clear which port they are aiming for, and second for all NHS workers – with all their very many complicated personal and work goals – to direct themselves **in general** to a common, agreed set of consistent ends.

I am optimistic enough to think that this is possible, despite all the political obstacles set against it. If you can bear with me for a few minutes longer I hope you will understand the reasons behind my unconventional approach to your problem. If, after this, you still think that my project is pointless we should call a halt to our meetings, and your Chairman can go ahead and shut the ward.

One of the ways in which I earn a living is to offer a 'personal analysis' service. I have found that some people find it therapeutic to try to examine their lives, purposes and behaviours in a more systematic way than they can on their own. One of my clients, Fred, is in a state not unlike the NHS.

Imagine this situation: one day Fred calls me to ask for a consultation. I discover that he is 45 and has, so far, managed to live a life without too much trauma. He has followed a conventional route in late 20th century Britain. He has a steady job, he has children, he has a comfortable house with the normal electronic gadgetry. Nevertheless he feels that there is something wrong with his life which he just cannot put his finger on. He seems to be making progress but he has a constant sense of unease. Can I help?

I agree to try, and I start with Fred rather in the way I began with you. I ask Fred: **what are your primary drives?** I talk with him, and give him time to think in private. After a while Fred writes down what he sees as his fundamental life goals. These are:

1. To secure the highest paid job he possibly can.
2. To have an open, caring, involved family life, with maximum 'quality time' with his wife and children.
3. To have a well-maintained home – ideally his goal is to redecorate it himself, outside and in, every two years.
4. To develop his understanding of life by studying at least one Higher Education course per year in his spare time.

Fred sums himself up as an ambitious, socially aware family man. But from my point of view, if these goals truly summarise the essential Fred, rather than the ideal suburban husband, I see a deeply confused, contradictory personality. No wonder he is uneasy, he gets by but he does so by trying to move in incompatible directions simultaneously.

As with the NHS, Fred's incompatible orientation is obvious enough: if he is constantly seeking financial reward (goal one) he will not be able to achieve goal two in full since, at the very least, he will be working long hours, and devising ways to move yet further up the ladder. If he genuinely strives for goal two he will find it very difficult to achieve life-goal three. Certainly he will find it difficult to do so without causing stress to himself and his family. Likewise, goal four seems, inescapably, to be in conflict with goal one since Fred does not have enough time for both.

What Fred finds is that he can achieve, or partly achieve, one or two of these goals but cannot have them all. Yet he has no doubt that he is living a rational life. I disagree with him but then I admit that I am probably looking for more consistency of purpose than contemporary Western culture usually allows. However, we manage to agree that it would be better if his life could make more sense to him, and we begin to explore options.

The simplest choice is for Fred to concentrate on one goal only, or on two at the most, and to abandon the others. But Fred is not happy about this, this is to ignore what life means to him. He says he has not come to me for that sort of simplistic advice. He wants to know how he can take these basic purposes and adapt them into something more coherent – into something which does fit together. He doesn't want my all-or-nothing logic because there is much more to his life than this, but he does want help to sort out some of the inner tensions and conflicts he feels.

I think that I might be able to help, and suggest that the way forward is to take each of his 'fundamental goals' in turn, and break them down into their constituent parts. Then we can decide which of these smaller parts makes the most sense, and which can be combined coherently with others. For instance, we may want to consider what Fred means by 'open', 'caring' and 'quality time' in his second goal.

Melanie: I'm not sure about all this. You are either saying something profound here, or you are making a painfully simple point.

Philosopher: I'm sorry if I'm stating the obvious, but I think we do need to be clear about my proposed method of investigation. The points I'm trying to draw out by discussing Fred and his situation are these. Firstly, in response to Simon's worry, I appreciate that logic and reason are not enough to sort out your problem by themselves. Unfortunately a great many of my professional colleagues do not share this view, and think that this sort of deliberation is sufficient on its own. This happens, for instance, when ethicists try to apply theoretical 'rules' and 'principles' to health care dilemmas without taking account of the more messy and unpredictable human factors which always surround such situations. It also happens, as you will see if you study my papers, when economists try to apply their logical models of the world to the world as it is – in so doing they tend to learn a lot more about the models than they do about the world itself.

Fred is like the NHS in his conflicting goals and complexity. Just as I proposed to do with Fred, I am prepared to try to dissect the 'four principles' to see if there is real sense lying within them. Of course, if Fred's life were to be laid out in this way then he would never again see himself in the same way, and so there is a danger that my client might collapse. This would be very damaging to Fred but in the case of the NHS it may be that this will not be such a bad thing.

Melanie: What happens if, even when the essential drives have been analysed, Fred's life still does not make sense?

Philosopher: In that case we will have to start afresh, and build up a set of drives with which he will feel easy, and which will stop his perpetual conflicts of purpose. If we can't find some ultimate justification for Fred, some basic drive which can help him resolve his conflicts, then he might just as well draw straws to decide what he should do in his life. One day he'll stay at home with his children, the next he'll work for 16 hours to make up for lost time.

Melanie: Are you taking this analogy all the way? Because if you are then you are suggesting that the NHS is just like a Fred with fundamentally incompatible essential drives. And if you are suggesting this then you are saying that our resource allocation decisions are actually **entirely** arbitrary – like sticking pins in a map at random.

Philosopher: If this is the way you think my arguments turn out then so be it. Of course it never feels this way to Fred because he has a host of rational drives within his 'boat', it is only when he bothers to work out where he is going and why he is going there that his activities begin to look arbitrary. It is up to you to decide whether the NHS is like this.

I think I can help you think the matter through, although I can't promise to offer a simple solution to your problem. If you want my help though you will have to take on a fair amount of reading. I have written one paper about each of the four principles of the NHS, and in so doing I have formed a view – which I doubt very much that you'll share – about the nature of the organisation as a whole. Each of the four papers tries to clarify the range of meanings each principle might have, and having done so indicates which of these carries the most weight. The first paper examines the notion of need.

Part Two: Four NHS Principles?

Paper Two

Need

District Health Authorities will be responsible for assessing the health needs of their populations and arranging for these needs to be met.

Hospitals and other units will be responsible for providing efficient and effective health services to meet the needs identified by health authorities.[31]

Introduction

Of the four supposed basic principles the assertion that the NHS should 'meet needs' seems the most definitive: people in need have problems, therefore a public service designed to eliminate need must be good. But although this would be true in a world where needs could be distinguished from other concerns without controversy, the world is not like this. In this world human activities are so complex that it is very difficult to identify need with certainty.

Once the question 'what is a need?' is taken seriously then what at first seems obvious very quickly becomes obscure. Is it, for instance, possible to make a firm distinction between a 'need' and a 'want'? If there is a difference, is a 'need' more important than a 'want' or vice versa? Should the health service be concerned with 'needs' as a priority? If it should, ought the NHS pay attention to generic 'human need', or should it concentrate upon a particular type of 'need'? And if it is correct for the health service to be selective about 'needs' should it seek first to meet 'medical needs', 'health needs', 'health care needs', or 'health service needs'? This highly abridged list of questions may appear abstract and possibly even irrelevant to some, but experience shows that where the philosophy of need is not taken seriously practical 'needs-assessment' tends to drift with the tide of fashion.

Since the late 1980s the government has required the health service to assess needs. In response health service managers have obediently implemented one programme of needs-assessment after another, with a resultant proliferation of health service jobs in the area. The job descriptions for these posts tend to be vague, specifying little more than that 'the employee shall assess the health needs of the community' and 'work to implement policies to meet these needs'. As a result the actual tasks undertaken by appointees tend to be disparate, varying in accordance with local factors and interests[32] – an inevitable consequence of the lack of a reasoned, practically specific definition of need. Definitions do exist in parts of the organisation but each is open to interpretation, and there are at least three to choose from. The most commonly occurring official versions are that:

1. Health care need is 'the ability to benefit from health care'.[33]
2. Health care need exists when there is 'ill health'.[34]
3. Health care need is a matter of expert judgement.[35]

Stability at a Cost

There is little doubt that all three definitions have been designed to ensure the maintenance of existing health service practices and priorities, rather than for their philosophical merit. Since the present proprietors of the NHS show no qualms about implementing tough practical measures to prohibit free speech[2,3] it is no surprise that they scorn philosophy. But although this may be one way to preserve the status quo, it nevertheless comes at a considerable price: whenever they do try to clarify a piece of policy-making they invariably end up in a hopeless muddle.

The Supply or Benefit Definition of Health Care Need

By way of introduction to this most characteristic health service phenomenon consider the centrally authorised statement that 'health care need' means the 'ability to benefit from health care'.[36] If this is true then useful health care services define what is needed by dint of their availability: or to put this more formally, the existence of effective treatment or care is a necessary condition for there to be a health care need.[37] It follows naturally from this view that the way to assess health needs is first to review services, and second to see how they can be 'targeted' most effectively – a move which leaves planners free to concentrate exclusively on the allocation of currently obtainable services. On this understanding of need there is no reason to compare existing services with potential alternatives, even though philosophical reflection on the goals of health work reveals a wide range of credible possibilities which might be tried out. Under the influence of the **benefit** definition, rather than begin with the neutral open question: **what does the population need most of all?** managers can ask: **how might our present and projected set of health care services be used to benefit the population, and so meet their health needs?** The first question requires analysis and policy-making from scratch, while the second adapts the meaning of need to match what is currently on offer. Although these questions may, superficially, appear fairly similar, they could hardly be more different. What is more, although this definition is 'state of the art' in the NHS, and can be used positively to redistribute badly managed resources, it has deep conceptual flaws which are readily exposed once 'the hidden agenda' is put to one side.

Expressed in full the supply or benefit definition of health care need says:

A person has a health care need if he or she is able to benefit from health care. Conversely, if a person is unable to benefit from health care then he or she does not have a health care need.

Spelt out like this it is extremely difficult to take the proposal seriously. It is one thing to say that a person has no need of useless services – but quite another to say that a person cannot need what she cannot have. The idea is nothing less than bizarre. It implies that:

1. If a person has HIV or AIDS then – in 'commonsense' – he has several health care needs. He may need palliative therapy, he will probably need advice on preventing infection, and he could certainly benefit from a cure. But – in 'NHSese' – the AIDS sufferer does not, and by definition cannot, need a cure. He cannot need one because no such thing exists. If a cure were to be available tomorrow, then he would have need of it. But not today.
2. If the existence of beneficial health care is a necessary condition for a person to have a health care need then:
    • In the past when there were less health services (assuming these to be the equivalent of health care) there was less health care need. And in the far past, when there were no useful health care services (if this ever was the case), there were no health care needs.
    • In the present, in the least prosperous nations where there are fewer health services, there are fewer needs for health care.
3. If health care need is defined only as the ability to benefit from health care, as health services expand, and as developments in medical technology and pharmaceuticals continue, so such increased provision 'creates need'. By definition, the more useful health services there are (even if they are only slightly useful), the more health care need there is. Consequently it is theoretically impossible to 'reduce need' by 'meeting it' with more services.

According to the supply definition, as what can be supplied changes so need changes – but this is 'looking-glass' logic – topsy-turvy and back to front. The definition has gained favour not because it makes any sense, but because it corresponds with what has happened to the NHS. It is popular simply because it fits in with what the NHS has become.

The Ill Health Definition of Health Care Need

According to this definition a health care need exists if and only if some deficiencies in a person's health exist which require medical care, but **can** exist whether or not a suitable treatment exists. So if a patient has an infection which requires treatment with antibiotics then it is correct to say that she needs the antibiotic, even if there are no antibiotics available. But if she does not know how to exercise properly, yet she is presently in normal health (as clinically defined) then she does not have a need of health care. She has a need only when she is in ill health.

The ill health view of health care need makes sense only within a health service system which perpetuates a restricted understanding of health. Only those cases of ill health which the system defines as its concern are said to need health service help. As with the supply definition, health care needs are defined by what the health care system has come to be and what it has come to do. At a stroke the definition limits the extent of the health service to the scope of medical services, and so helps ensure that the health service continues to supply predominantly medical treatments and expertise.

Apparently the supply and ill health definitions support themselves nicely. Where the ill health approach runs into problems (for example, it cannot by itself talk of 'the need for health promotion services') the supply definition offers solutions (if 'health promotion' is a beneficial health care service currently provided then it must be needed). But this restrictive and incestuous arrangement is permissible only if it is assumed that what the NHS does sets limits on what health needs there can be in the real world, which of course it does not.

The Normative Definition of Health Care Need

The normative definition is:

> . . . the idea that health care need is a matter of opinion. The identity of the assessor is included in the definition, and whether a health care need exists or not depends on the needs of the assessor.[38]

On this explanation needs do not necessarily depend upon what is supplied, nor necessarily on the presence of ill health. Whether or not these conditions apply, need can be brought into being by expert judgement. In this way a need for health care can come about when an assessor believes that health care ought to be provided. For example, if a health service planner has decided that screening services should be offered to a particular target group then it will follow that the group has a need of health care. Conversely, once an expert decision has been made that people over a certain age should not be screened then it must follow that this group does not have a need for health care.

Normative judgements about need are made constantly in the health service. Every time a doctor makes a decision to prescribe or not she is both 'assessing need' and acting on her judgement. Without such judgements it is hard to see how the health service, or indeed any professional service, could function. But just because normative judgements are often required for practice this does not necessarily mean that they are always appropriate or best. Firstly, the 'expert' can be wrong. Indeed it is quite normal for 'experts' to differ widely in their judgements about what is needed.[39,40] Secondly, the 'expert's' perception of what is needed can be different from the recipient's view. Normative needs-assessment can offer no help in resolving such differences, other than to be of use in 'technical support' of the belief that the patient is mistaken. Thirdly, in common with the other NHS definitions of need, normative judgements reinforce the status quo. And of the three, the normative definition is the most blatant. It makes it quite explicit that those who the health service designates as experts are entitled not only to assess needs, but also actually to say what needs there are in the first place (an example of this would occur where a doctor opposed to the practice of osteopathy prescribes a pain-killer for soreness caused by poor posture, and rules out manipulation). And as the 'experts' do this, so it is probable that more of the services which they judge necessary will be supplied. And if (as is normal) the assessors are expert in ill-health as medically defined, the nature of what is supplied will reflect that knowledge, and those interests. And so it goes on. Each NHS definition offers support to the others, even though they cannot logically be used simultaneously in every case. And each is deeply orthodox, protecting and preserving the current status of the NHS, whatever it is at a particular time.

Chains in the Wall

For those who would change the NHS these definitions of need can seem like chains hammered into a dungeon wall. They allow some movement, and may even allow a lot of freedom to those who get used to them, but they do not allow captives to leave their confines. Inside the health service 'needs language' is not used in the same way as in the world beyond. Perhaps the differences in meaning are only slight, but the more subtle they are the more difficult it can be to achieve a distance from them.

However, despite their strength, the chains can be cut with the right tools. Analysis of the three NHS definitions of health care need reveals that:

1. 'Needs-assessment' is controversial. Alternative definitions of health care need co-exist, and the 'right' one is not obvious. Choices have to be made, and so require justification by those who use them and take them seriously within the health service: Which needs? Whose needs? Who says?
2. Each definition limits the range of need which it claims the NHS should address, and does so without philosophical justification.
3. Each definition is seriously flawed. Yet if need is to be used as a criterion for rationing health care (which is often suggested), then rational analysis, from as objective a perspective as possible, is surely morally required. If need is to be used as a NHS tool then, just as with drug dosages and machine specifications, technical accuracy should be a required standard. On the other hand, if 'needs assessment' is an inherently vague procedure then the nature of this vagueness must be clearly demonstrated. If there is more than one way to assess need, then openness about any underlying reasoning is imperative. If needs assessment is an obscure process, what is it hiding?
4. Since none of the definitions stem from independent analysis, but are based instead on contingent service provision and what experts deem to be necessary, and since actual practice is an amalgamation of contradictory purposes, official needs-assessment cannot help but be an inconsistent process.

A Philosophical Approach

If need is to be genuinely understood, if its meaning is to be discovered rather than invented, then all preconditions and practicalities must, temporarily at least, be put to one side. In particular, thinking about need must not be coloured by the present set-up of the NHS. The fact that strong traditions and practices have been established over the years has nothing whatsoever to do with the quest for a sound definition of need. Rigorous open-minded thinking is indispensable, and this thinking must take place independently of the drives and processes of the NHS. However uncomfortable the results may turn out to be, philosophical inquiry into the nature of need must – as far as this is possible – remain unpolluted by outside influence.

Need as Fundamental

A popular view, among philosophers and non-philosophers alike, is that there is something special about needs.[41] The idea that need is an exceptional category, that needs are somehow fundamental and basic to human interests, is widespread and compelling. The doctrine that 'human need should be met' has such emotive force that arguments in defence of the NHS frequently rest on an ultimate, though vague appeal to it. At rock-bottom many feel that if needs are neglected then everything else of moral importance is neglected too.

This contention has many forms, of which this is one:

> In a cynical society, in a society where devotion to consumerism and competition freely permits aggression and attack, and where it is praiseworthy to benefit at the expense of others – even to the point where they may be ruined – one standard still remains. This is, that as a matter of fact people have needs. Some of these needs are essential to their flourishing, some are essential to their very existence. If these basic needs are not satisfied – if people are denied food, shelter, hope, education, medicine, security, and the chance to develop – then this is unquestionably immoral. If the price of competition between people is that many do not even have their elementary needs guaranteed, then any semblance of morality disappears.

Of contemporary philosophical work the writing of Garrett Thomson is the most forthright in its support for the view of need as a special, distinct category. For Thomson need is the root of all morality. Of all the words political philosophers find interesting, need is in a class of its own. It might be possible to debate endlessly about the true nature of liberty, or about the most just organisation of society, but it is not right to argue about the set of basic needs. These needs just are. Thomson's thesis is that the 'concept of need' forces recognition of what we are morally required to do, and so boils moral debate down to basics. Whenever fundamental needs are detected then, as far as Thomson is concerned, it is undeniable that they ought to be met. Far from being a 'rhetorical device', as some people think:

> Needs are objectives in the sense that it is a discoverable matter of fact what needs people have and this fact has an intrinsic bearing on what we ought to do. 'Need' allows us to pass from an 'is' statement to an 'ought'.[42]

Thomson reinforces this claim by opposing a view that needs are nothing more than requirements for other ends. He denies that all needs are 'instrumental' on the ground that some things are needed for their own sake. Serious damage results if these needs are not met, which is bad in itself. He describes those things which it would be disastrous or damaging to lack as 'normative' or 'fundamental' needs, and offers examples:

> Britain needs the fresh start of the Alliance [a now defunct British political party]; I need your love; this child needs food.[42] (My parentheses.)

Party politics aside Thomson's point is that the unloved person and the hungry child can – purely and simply – be said to need love and food respectively since without these essentials they must be disastrously harmed. In Thomson's opinion it is superfluous to say that these things are needed **for** something else – they are needed, full stop. He is thoroughly opposed to the idea that needs make sense only in relation to prior purposes, for if this were so it would be no use pointing to basic unmet needs as immoral facts – facts which must be improved if morality is to succeed. And without this, he adds, what is left of morality?

Need as a Gap

The Swedish philosopher Per-Erik Liss also regards need as an important category, and suggests that by ranking needs, progress may be made towards the fairer rationing of scarce health care resources. However, he does not believe that needs can be thought of as 'immoral facts', or as 'fundamental'. For Liss need is most simply thought of as a **gap** or a **difference**. Nothing more. He argues that there are two conditions necessary for a need to exist:

1. There must be a gap between the actual state (AS) and the goal (G).
2. If X is necessary to achieve G (or in other words 'to fill the gap') then there is a need for X.[43]

Put this simply the conditions look inescapably obvious, and hardly seem worth stating. But they are essential to an unprejudiced understanding of need, and are habitually overlooked by those involved in the NHS version of needs-assessment. However, through his philosophical instinct and determination to understand the world rather than design it Liss recognises their importance. His insistence that need is essentially the gap between AS and G is crucial since it disentangles the notion of need both from people's opinion about what is needed, and from any connection with health services and 'states of illness'. Liss' analysis purifies need, removing the contaminants of convention and human politics through a process of philosophical distillation.

Liss also emphasises that it is a profound mistake to think of needs as objects. Needs exist when the two necessary conditions exist, but needs are not physical things. If they were, and you were in possession of the object, you could then still be said to 'have a need'. So, to be given the food you need would then give you the need itself, which would be silly. For Liss the only logical way in which to think of food, in this case, would be as follows.

If AS = hunger; G = well fed; X = food, and a person is hungry, then there is a need for X in order to achieve G. X itself is not the need. The need should be understood as the combination of what is missing (when a person is in need) and what is necessary to fill up 'the hole' (when something is needed).

Liss' insistence on clarifying these most basic of points can be a little hard to appreciate. But what he shows, by demonstrating that need is a gap and needs are not simple objects, is that it is just incorrect to talk of medicines and medical technology as unquestionable needs. These things can be said to be needed only if there is a gap between the actual state of a person and the goal to be achieved, and only if they fill it. In other words, unlike the NHS account of needs assessment which is bound to support whatever arrangements are in place at a certain time, Liss' approach constantly forces critical examination of whether things are needed or not.

Need as Instrumental

In contrast to the three NHS definitions of need this alternative holds that rather than shape definition in accord with what now exists (either as a health service, an illness, or an external point of view) the key to understanding need is to ask, 'what state or goal is sought by the individual?' This view includes states which are intentionally sought – for example, where a person seeks advice to help herself quit smoking; and states which are of benefit but not sought psychologically – for example, where the body of a baby rids itself, unintentionally, of infection. Whatever means are necessary to achieve the goal then become those things which are needed.

Liss prefers this definition because it makes logical sense. It explains why something must be said to be a need, without presupposing the limits of need. What is needed obviously depends upon purpose (and, of course, the fact that the NHS lacks a theory of purpose partially accounts for its idiosyncratic use of needs language):

> There will be no need at all if there is no goal to have a need for. It seems odd to answer the question 'why do you need X?' with 'for no reason at all, I just need it'. Let us use our imagination and think of a person in a situation where there are no goals . . . (I admit it is difficult). In this case the person has no needs, nor needs anything. But someone might insist and say, 'At least he needs to eat'. 'Why?' 'He will die'. 'Certainly, and there is the goal'. The need to eat exists only if there is such a goal as to live. No such goal, no need to eat.[44]

Liss thinks further that:

> A person has a need of health care when (a) there is a difference between the actual state and the technical state of health and (b) health care is necessary in order to attain the technical state of health.[45]

However, although this may be philosophically neat, and clearly valid in the abstract, it leaves all practical questions untouched. If needs can only be understood instrumentally then what is needed is, on every occasion, defined by purpose. But without specifying purpose – in this case without saying what the 'technical state of health' is – there can be no practical specification of need.

Further Clarification

In order to establish a positive view of the nature of need, and so gain a grasp of the real extent of this 'health service principle', as many potential misunderstandings as possible must be cleared away.

Needs are not Objective Facts

Although it is a matter of fact that members of the human species need oxygen in order to live, it does not follow that even something as basic as oxygen is objectively and always a human need. The fact that an element is essential to life does not mean that it is therefore needed in all cases. Needs are not brute facts but are dependent upon purpose. Since breathing is an essential part of human existence, oxygen is a strong candidate for the title 'objective need'. But biological survival – the continuing operation of the body's pre-programming – is not the only human purpose possible, nor is it obviously an overriding purpose.

What is needed is not necessarily fixed but can change as other factors change. Although oxygen is needed by human beings for most of the time, it is not always needed. According to circumstances other needs might be greater. For example, a person might be in great pain, terminally ill, and elect for euthanasia to avoid harm. Or life may become unbearable and a person may need to commit suicide, and so choose to feed exhaust fumes into a sealed car. Reflection shows that any candidate for the title 'objective need' can be overridden as conditions alter and opinion changes.

Garrett Thomson has suggested that 'self-respect' is an example of a permanent, unshakeable need. He says:

> If a man must suffer serious harm so long as he lacks self-respect, then he has a need of self-respect. Such a need is non-instrumental in that it relates to the overall quality of a person's life rather than to a particular goal he happens to have. This kind of non-instrumental need I call a 'fundamental need'.[46]

However, whatever thing, event, or process is said to be a 'fundamental need', there will always be occasions on which it is not. For instance, it may be necessary for a person to lose self-respect (to do something he finds degrading) in order to survive to fight another day. For instance it is a sad fact that some people find that they have to be bowed and subservient in order to protect their positions at work. And some women are placed in a position (which they do not want) where they have no alternative but to turn to prostitution to earn money.

What is more, some people sometimes respect themselves when they are not entitled to do so. We may continue to have self-respect when we are behaving shabbily, in which case self-respect stands in the way of our noticing our faults. In such a case it can plausibly be said that the more basic need is to recognise and change our faults, and not for self-respect.

Indeed self-respect might just as well be called a 'multi-instrumental need', in that self-respect is needed to allow the doing of a great many things (but not all things) which are important to a person. Self-respect may well be crucial to an individual, but if it is it will be crucial for reasons of function – it will be essential to allow other good things to happen.

The Avoidance of Harm does not Guarantee that Something is Needed

The avoidance of harm, and there being a need for something, are often related. But the fact that harm has been avoided does not guarantee that a 'fundamental need has been met'.[41] If a person does not have the means to achieve something, and will be harmed by this lack (and may even be seriously harmed by it) then this is certainly an indication that the need or lack in question is important (and may even be very important). However, just as it is not possible to point to needs as 'objective facts' so it is not possible to:

1. Identify a simple and fixed list of objective harms.
2. Say with certainty that what is harm for one person is also harmful to another.
3. Say that a clear and steady ranking of harms exists.

It is often assumed that 'harm' and 'need' are inevitably linked, but this is not true. In fact a person can often need something without suffering harm if he lacks it. For example, I might need a computer disc in order to work on my book, and I might have left it at home, so being unable to work on the disc is a prima-facie harm. However, it does not follow that I am truly harmed by this so long as I do something else which I also need to do. In other words, **so long as there are other beneficial possibilities open to a person then harm and need are not necessarily associated – it is only when there are no other ways forward that this is the case**. The loss of my needed disc is not a harm if, for instance, I go for a fulfilling walk with my wife, or work on a harder section of the book in longhand. Indeed, the lack of a particular thing which is needed may well produce more benefit than harm, even though one sort of harm would have been avoided if the need had been met.

The essential point about harm is not that harm is bad full stop, but that harm is bad because of what it prevents people from doing. The notion of harm makes sense only if something good is prevented – the more serious the harm the greater the potential good impeded. Harm makes sense only in relation to a beneficial purpose stopped. Consequently, the only way it makes real sense to think of needs is in relation to action – needs must be thought of in terms of **what is required** – what is required for the next second, minute or lifetime? What is required for the time ahead?

Needs and Wants are Hardly Ever Separate Categories

If it is the case that need (i.e. the lack of something) can be understood in practice only as 'a lack of means' then any means to a beneficial end can properly be described as needed. However, out of convention and the wish not to describe something as 'really that important', on many occasions the word 'want' is preferred instead. For example, Thomson has written:

> Consider first the simple equivalence 'A needs X' = 'A wants X'. This equivalence fails to hold in either direction. For (a) we often say of people that they want things which they do not need, for instance, a child who demands a lollipop . . . certainly wants a lollipop, but we are most unlikely to acknowledge that he needs one, (b) we (rather less often) say of people that they need things which they do not want, e.g. to eat more health food.[47]

But the child described might well have had a reason for his demand – for instance, he might have wanted to feel refreshed and calm on a summer's day. And if he had a reason (to be refreshed and calm) then it is correct to say that he needed the lollipop.

The Importance of Purpose

The view that 'needs' override 'wants' can be sustained only if it is possible to establish that there is such a category as 'fundamental need', and it has been seen that this cannot be done.* Instead an unbreakable link between needs and purpose has been revealed, and this in turn emphasises the fundamental importance of establishing the best health service purpose or set of purposes – before engaging in needs-assessment. When someone says 'I need food' and another says 'I want food' there may or may not be a difference in kind, and the way to establish this is not to establish once and for all that food is a fundamental need but to look at each case and discover what the food will do. If one person is starving and the other is fat then it will be more important to feed the hungry man, and this remains the case regardless of the words we use to describe the situation (even if it were the starving man who had said 'I want food' one would still feed him in preference to the obese one, even if the fat man claimed to need the food). The answer does not rest with the use of language but with **what the giving of the food to one man rather than another makes possible.** The important thing is to look to see what aspects of life are enabled by the means rather than at whether a given state is one of wanting rather than needing.

Per-Erik Liss argues that the idea of 'want' is not equivalent to 'need', and does so for the technical reason that a 'want' is not the same sort of thing as 'the gap' he writes of. Unless used as synonymous with 'a lack', a 'want' is not Liss' gap since 'wanting' is a question of desire, and is a psychological state. The objects necessary to meet need and want can be the same but 'want' and 'need' are not the same – 'want' is formulated and reasoned – needs are just gaps.

This distinction has important implications, particularly in the field of 'health promotion', where many seek a justification for intervening in other people's lives according to 'health promotion values' rather than the subject's

---

* This is not to say that it is *unreasonable*, either in theory or practice, to argue for the provision of means which meet the most important needs of almost all people almost all of the time. Indeed, such an argument is part of the basis of my own theory of health.

values. For example, the many 'health promoters' who endeavour to persuade people to drink less may find support in Liss' account. For Liss (and his colleague Nordenfelt) it is theoretically possible to want two bottles of liquor in the morning but not need them. The argument is that one might have a psychological desire for these things but need (i.e. *really* need) to go to work, to paint the house, or to do some other more constructive activity.

But this argument will not hold up. If a person wants X then almost always she must have a reason for wanting X, and if she then does not do anything about getting X this shows only that she wants something else more. In other words it may be that a person has better reasons for something else (so she might need the liquor to get drunk, or happy, but might need her wages more). One might say 'Oh, I want to smoke but I don't need to . . .' by which one might well mean that it is not necessary to smoke. But what this really means is:

> I am in a particular state at this time and I have a number of possible goals. I particularly need to relax and I can achieve this goal equally well either by smoking or jogging. To achieve G I can fill the gap either by going out for a run or lighting a cigarette. Thus it makes as much sense to say that I need a cigarette as it does to say that I need to go for a run. I enjoy smoking and running and I desire both. However, the reason I jog rather than smoke is because jogging allows me to achieve further goals which smoking does not – but technically it is right to say that I need to smoke to achieve my goal.

The Biological Trap

There is a yet more basic reason why the view that 'needs should override desires' should not be accepted without question. If it is believed that non-reasoned needs are more basic than reasoned wants (and for the very reason that they are not thought about) then we fall into the trap of accepting that because biological needs (or the unconscious/programmed human life goals) are 'fundamental' then action to provide these needs must take priority over other possible needs. And this is to fall into the trap of accepting a 'medical model' of health care, of accepting the category mistake that disease and health are on a single continuum,[48] and of accepting that those in control of medical care can always override reasoned choice on the ground of biological protection (you might think you need to go home but what you really need is . . .!!). Even if every expert in the world agrees that you need to have your 'Xectomy' this is not a binding reason to force you to have it, provided that you are not generally deluded and know what you need.

What Needs Are

As has been seen, it is possible to think of a need as simply a gap between two different states of being – one actual and the other potential. Need then means the lack of something, as a pauper is said to be in need of money. However, at one stage beyond this purist approach, needs are best regarded as means towards ends. Practically, the pauper needs money to achieve certain goals. Everything that can properly be called a need is not a 'need in itself' (it makes no sense to say of something that it is a 'means in itself'). Anything needed must be needed for something else to happen. All needs must have ends or targets, although it is not necessary for these ends or targets to be consciously selected. If purposes change – however they change – then needs change too.

Needs and wants might be pictured in the following way – a thing, a procedure, an event, or a change can be:

1. *Wanted only* (wanted and not needed)
   This category includes things which are not necessary, things which are not means, things which are not required for any real purpose. Actual examples are not easy to imagine, but might be such frivolous desires as wanting the very best car wash when another sort would get the car equally clean, or wanting a haircut despite having had a perfectly adequate one the day before. Also in this category are things which are sought after as the result of a mistaken belief, or a delusion. For instance, a person may believe he needs a haircut simply because he has forgotten that he had one yesterday. Someone may believe that she needs a course of drugs (and so want those drugs) when the evidence is that they will do her no good or will even do harm. A woman may believe that her neighbour's answering machine is sexually molesting her and want it restrained – but this is hardly what she needs. Or you may just have a whim to walk down a country lane, for no reason you understand, and then wonder why you are there because you are gaining no benefit from the activity: **when something is wanted and not needed the touchstone is that no benefit is to be obtained from the desire**.

   The category is not clear-cut however. There are borderline cases. For instance, if I say 'I need a Diet Tango' I may just be expressing a trivial desire if all I want is any fizzy drink. And in common language it seems an unnecessary exaggeration to say that a Diet Tango is needed since it is unlikely to be a consideration of much importance. However, if I have a purpose which requires a Diet Tango then, technically, I must say that 'I need (and want) a Diet Tango'. If for instance I have been exercising and I have found that only Diet Tango is truly refreshing after exercise, then the Diet Tango is a means towards my refreshment, and in this case I can quite correctly say that I need it.

2. *Needed only* (needed but not desired)
   Examples in this category may be taken from a sizeable part of the spectrum (see Fig. 3). All that is necessary to qualify is that something is a means towards an end which can benefit a person, and the person does not (for whatever reason) recognise the need, or does not have any psychological desire to have whatever it is. Actual examples might include education for a youth (not always recognised as needed by young people) or vitamins for a person who does not know what these are (again, not recognised by the person), or oxygen, or food (for the unconscious patient). This section can include not only apparently fundamental things but also things as simple as a drink for a baby, a sheet smoothed on a bed for a patient who is not comfortable but does not know why, or a window opened to relieve a headache (not thought of, and even positively not wanted by a person who

does not like the cold – but who does not recognise that he is being harmed to a greater extent by his headache). So, in this category it is possible to need things and not want them because:

- They are not known.
- It is not recognised that the thing is needed.
- The end is not recognised to be beneficial (prior to its achievement).

3. *Wanted and needed*

Potentially everything can be both wanted and needed. All that is required is sufficient knowledge to allow the identification and recognition of all needs, and also reasons to assert that the things other people might trivialise as wants are actually needed. In other words what is required is that we can say why this thing counts as a means for us. Or, alternatively, if we are advocating for others, how this thing counts as a means for them. It is possible that a person will have a reason for even the most trivial thing, yet will not be able to make himself understood to you.

4. *Needed and not wanted* (positively shunned although clear benefit is possible)

This is a very important section because it allows for the assertion of will in cases where others might insist that what they perceive to be 'needed' should take precedence.[48,49] For example, a person may need chemotherapy to cure her of her cancer, yet she may not want it. Alternatively, a person might be defined as needing screening for disease but might not want it, and so reject it. In such cases other goals, and therefore other needs, will be defined by the subject as being of greater importance. For instance, relaxation therapy, pain management, or simply being at home with the family and not being treated medically at all, might be preferred to chemotherapy.

(3) In principle, all means can be needed and wanted	
(1) Wanted only – not needed	(2) Needed only – without desire
(4) Needed and not wanted – positively shunned Will is asserted by the subject. In this case 'instrumental need' defined by the potential recipient of health services takes precedence over other types	

Fig. 2

Means towards the most trivial of ends, e.g. "I need a Diet Tango". Such statements are usually said as wants, in common language. However, such statements properly and correctly describe needs if they refer to means necessary to achieve a beneficial goal

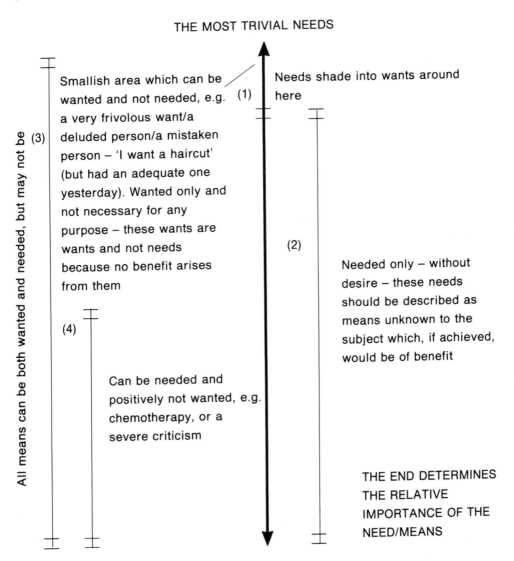

THE MOST TRIVIAL NEEDS

Smallish area which can be wanted and not needed, e.g. (1) a very frivolous want/a deluded person/a mistaken person – 'I want a haircut' (but had an adequate one yesterday). Wanted only and not necessary for any purpose – these wants are wants and not needs because no benefit arises from them

Needs shade into wants around here

(3)

(2)

Needed only – without desire – these needs should be described as means unknown to the subject which, if achieved, would be of benefit

(4)

All means can be both wanted and needed, but may not be

Can be needed and positively not wanted, e.g. chemotherapy, or a severe criticism

THE END DETERMINES THE RELATIVE IMPORTANCE OF THE NEED/MEANS

THE MOST IMPORTANT NEEDS
(if these are not met the subject will have very little, or even no autonomy)

"I need a life-saving op", "I need hope", "I need self-respect", "I need a home", "I need information", "I need to understand my situation".

Fig. 3

Review

What is Clear so Far

First of all it must be stressed that none of this analysis, and especially none of the criticism of contemporary needs-assessment, is meant to imply that assessing need is not important. The trouble is that there are so many different types of need, and so many different perspectives from which need can be assessed (and it is undeniable that assessments from different perspectives can produce different accounts of what is needed), that it is essential first of all to be clear about **why** needs-assessment is so important, and which of the indefinite range of needs is the most important set to meet. And at present these matters are not clear.

It may, however, be provisionally concluded that:

1. It is very difficult even to define 'a need' in the abstract, never mind to be authoritative about actual needs.
2. At least three different definitions of 'health care need' or 'health need' are currently maintained within the NHS.
3. Of the three definitions it is not clear which is the priority for the NHS. And what is more there are no rules available to help those in charge of the organisation to decide.
4. Present definitions of need in the NHS start from 'what is' rather than 'what could be'. What is more they assume, within their structure, that a clear and agreed health service purpose exists (which is not true). This lack of clear purpose is indicated even by the NHS definitions of need themselves, since each implies a number of possible purposes which are incompatible when taken together.
5. Each definition is philosophically problematic, and each is far too weak to guide consistent, specific policy-making.
6. Philosophical analysis shows that need can only be generally and neutrally understood as 'instrumental'. It also demonstrates that need is not an overriding arbiter, nor is it a basic single principle which can be applied to solve the rationing problems of the health service.
7. All three definitions take little or no account of the user's perspective on what is needed (because none is explicitly instrumental). Thus, the instrumental account of need is to be preferred since it requires the clearest specification of purpose, demands that potential benefits can be demonstrated, and allows subjects to be involved in needs-assessment (whereas the NHS definitions preclude participation).

This is not to say that the instrumental version of needs-assessment is the best alternative in every case, nor that the other definitions are totally flawed – they are merely limited. Of the official definitions, although it might be the most limiting of all in the wrong hands, the normative definition of need can be used wisely and may form part of the best health care practice so long as it is remembered that it is not the only legitimate definition.

Summary: What Needs Are

Needs exist only if goals exist – needs are means to ends (needs must therefore ultimately always be understood as instrumental)

There is no need if no potential benefit can be had

Ends govern needs, in this ranking:

1. Ends
2. Needs

Need and harm are not inevitably linked

The notion of harm makes sense only in relation to a goal or purpose prevented

There is a vital difference between a) the approach which works by meeting need guided by what exists, and b) the approach which specifies the goals or purposes sought. The difference is vision

Consequently needs should be assessed not according to whether they are fundamental or not, but according to the extent to which their satisfaction makes **beneficial doing** possible (see also p. 92, autonomy as the basic cost)

It is a serious error to claim that 'reasoned wants' are inferior to 'non-reasoned needs' because:

1. There is no absolute distinction between needs and wants
2. The assertion places biological or medical purposes above other purposes – it produces biological imperatives. If these imperatives are then said to be health needs the biological trap is sprung

Fig. 4

Paper Three

Quality

PART ONE

During the 1980s the idea that health services should be the 'best available'[15] changed into the apparently similar phrase, 'health care services should be quality services'. But despite appearances, the contemporary understanding of 'quality service' is quite different from that of 'best service', as this paper will demonstrate.

A Principle 'Evolves'

Throughout the last decade, and with increasing enthusiasm into the 1990s, the NHS adopted a fashionable 'philosophy of quality' from the business world.* By 1989 the Department of Health was officially encouraging a 'managed approach to quality' in the NHS, a policy which was formally extended in 1990 to cover 23 sites, including some whole districts.[50] Even though the differences between running a profit-making business and offering a caring service are widely acknowledged, such slogans as 'quality assurance', 'total quality management' and 'quality circles' have become common currency in the health service.[51] Numerous staff are now part or fully employed to research and monitor quality (or to 'audit'[52]), while many others write occasional documents which attempt to explain what 'quality' is, and how the health service might achieve more of it. There is even a journal, launched by BMA Publishing in 1992, devoted solely to *Quality in Health Care*.**

However, in order to have a policy to produce 'quality health care' it is necessary, at the very least, for there to be clarity about what 'quality health care' is. If nothing else a philosophically sound distinction between 'quality health care' and plain ordinary 'non-quality health care' is required, and for this a proper analysis of 'quality' *per se* is essential. In the absence of a lucid and practical definition the word lies open to manipulation by any interest group which lays claim to it. Yet, just as is the case with need, despite its extensive use in health service literature, no one acting for the NHS has yet developed a convincing account of quality.

---

* The NHS has also been influenced by 'health systems analysis' in the US, much of which advocates 'quality assurance'.
** There is a *Quality Review Bulletin* in the US.

Analysing Quality

Before embarking on detailed analysis of the meaning of 'quality', and the unusual use of this term in the NHS, it is worth noting that normally when something is said to be 'quality' the intention is to describe that thing favourably: 'this house has quality', 'that academic has quality written all over her'. However it is useful to bear in mind that 'quality' does not have to be 'good'. Certainly things are very often said to be of 'good quality', but may equally properly be described as 'poor' or 'appalling' quality. Nonetheless, unless an adjective has been added it is safest to assume (at least in everyday life, outside the world of commerce and modern health care) that when something is described as 'being of quality' the implication is that it is a thing of high calibre.

Definitions from Commerce

To seek to supply quality products and services is an established feature of business language and management. The basic idea – which features in every textbook – is that any decent business ought to be producing and selling 'quality goods' while keeping costs to a minimum. Consequently the literature either defines quality in a way which incorporates cheapness, or which necessarily associates quality with the willingness of the customer to purchase.

The following 'definitions' of quality are representative of the genre. They may be found in various textbooks on commercial management (and all appear in Oakland's book *TQM*):

1. **The totality of features and characteristics of a product or a service that bear on its ability to satisfy stated or implied needs**[53] (the British Standard 'definition').

Scrutiny of this statement reveals that despite its intent it is not a definition of quality at all. Translated into more accessible English it says:

'Quality is a product or service which may or may not satisfy needs'.

In other words, absolutely any product or service may be said to be quality according to the British Standard, which renders the ascription of 'quality' quite redundant. More generously, the phrase is probably intended to mean something like this:

'A quality product or service has characteristics which satisfy the needs of customers'.

Although still not a definition of quality, this statement implies that any service which 'satisfies customer needs' must count as a quality service. However, even if this is what the 'British Standard definition' is supposed to mean it is so ambiguous that it fails to offer any explanation of what quality is. It does provide one elementary way to gauge successful manufacture or service provision, but it says nothing about quality outside the limited context of the commercial transaction.

Quality is not 'Qualities'

The type of commercial definition which emphasises 'characteristics' and 'features' confuses 'quality' with 'qualities'. Such an approach fails to understand that the fact that a product must have at least one 'desired quality' in order to sell does not mean that the product must therefore be **of** quality.

In commerce there is a natural reluctance to set absolute 'quality standards' since to do so may act to restrict profit margins. If an organisation's essential purpose is to make as much money as possible it is better to link quality to 'sellability' rather than to have to discard unnecessarily those products which fall below pre-set 'quality standards'. But, financial prudence apart, such simple pragmatism is not sufficient to provide a sound definition. In copying an approach from business those employed in 'quality assurance' in the health service have taken an identical line, and so have reproduced the same conceptual error. To give one example, in a recently produced NHS training pack[54] under the heading 'What is Quality?' it is said that:

> Quality can be taken to refer to those attributes or characteristics of a service which are valued by people with an interest in the service.

The sentiment has moved from the world of selling to the world of health care, and 'valued' has been substituted for 'needed', but still the amended statement fails to define quality (meaningful definitions do not timidly 'refer' to things, they explain them). Instead it equates 'quality' as a general idea with 'qualities' as attributes or characteristics of things. But any product or service, however poor, will have 'attributes'. Whether they are regarded as 'good', 'bad' or 'indifferent' – whether they are valued or not – these attributes may, nevertheless, be correctly described as 'qualities'. One person might well describe the 'attribute' in question as a 'good quality' or a 'desirable quality' whilst another might describe it as a 'bad' or an 'undesirable quality' without fundamental contradiction. Such evaluations can be quite separate from judgements about the quality **of** something. It is quite possible for a person to say 'I think that this is a poor quality', meaning 'I do not value this attribute', yet at the same time to admit that the quality of the attribute is good. For example, one might quite properly argue that a 'managed approach' to health care is not a 'desired quality' whilst confessing that the standard of management is high. Equally, it is possible to regard an 'attribute' or 'quality' of something as valuable, yet simultaneously confess that it is not 'of good quality'. It may be, for example, that a person always becomes involved in the decision-making of a committee (and this involvement is a 'quality' she has), yet her contributions are consistently intellectually weak. In such a case the 'quality' in question is not up to the required cognitive level, and so is said not to be of quality, even though the person's involvement is valued nonetheless.

So, to say that 'quality can be taken to refer to those attributes which are valued by those with an interest in the service' is inadequate on three counts:

1. It is not a definition.
2. No overt standard (other than the preferences of anyone 'with an interest',

however well or ill informed) is set by which to judge quality. Thus, according to this view quality must vary relative to what people value or even, if choice is limited, what they are prepared to accept (which, of course, is the main reason why some NHS policy-makers are trying to re-model 'quality'). Different 'customers' will accept different levels of service – some people will tolerate far longer waiting times to see a doctor than others – some will 'value' a 20-minute wait as reasonable, others will complain.

If a service is very poor by normal standards, if, for example, only the most basic medical equipment is available (as in Sarajevo throughout most of 1992–93) then people may still value even these most rudimentary facilities. In this way quality becomes not intrinsic to things but changes according to 'consumer tolerance', which means that the quality of something can be driven down during recession or when resources are scarce. On this understanding of quality **any** food will be quality food for a starving person, but will not count as quality food in the eyes of the well-fed vegetarian. On this account when there has been no medicine any medicine may be valued as better than nothing. But this comprehensively weakens the meaning of quality, transforming an important idea into a notion which can change with the wind.

3. There may be considerable differences in the perception of a giver and receiver of the same service – both of whom could properly be said to have an interest in it. For instance a doctor might well value the salary structure of the NHS whereas his patient might take a different view, judging (albeit in political innocence) that lower wages for doctors would mean more resources for himself, and for other patients. Without doubt 'the rate of pay for clinicians is an attribute valued by (at least some of) those with an interest in the service', but it is absurd to argue from this that therefore the salary structure must be a 'quality salary structure'. All that can be said is that the structure is a 'quality' valued by some and that it is, at the same time a 'quality' not valued by others. Clearly, quality in the usual sense of the word is not at issue within this strange account.

These criticisms are not meant to condemn the general intention to identify quality with the interests of the users of the health service (a view which is basically in harmony with the requirement to involve subjects in establishing their instrumental needs). The problem lies not in the motivation but in the lack of sustained philosophical spadework. The real challenge is to translate this belief – in the importance of taking seriously the views of all those with an interest in the NHS – into a weighty argument. As things stand there are two flawed assumptions to be dealt with, beyond the lack of definition. Firstly (via roots in commerce), it is assumed that users of a national health service in which there is little or no real competition for their patronage, are able to express their interests through their behaviour as if they were prospective automobile buyers. Secondly, it is taken for granted that the act of 'valuing' a service is done from an informed position, which is often not the case. However, such a condition must surely apply if 'valuing' is to have any real meaning.

2. Quality is simply meeting the requirements of the customer[53]

Like 'definition' 1 this explanation regards quality as free floating – something which, like everything else in an open market, will find its own level. Furthermore it fails to suggest any means by which to judge what quality truly is in cases where the 'requirements of customers' conflict (either with those of the provider, or – especially in scarcity – with those of other customers).

3. The object of quality control is to produce a quality that:
- Satisfies the customer
- Is as cheap as possible
- Can be achieved in time to meet delivery requirements.[55]

For fear that the above definition may seem too dry it might be substituted for this more popular alternative:

> 'We know that the gun we have supplied is a quality weapon because Mr Capone is happy with his purchase. He says it satisfies his needs. Mr Capone is very choosy but we were able to supply him at lowest cost. And we had one in stock, so delivery was instantaneous'.

4. A predictable degree of uniformity and dependability at low cost and suited to the market.[56]

The above two interpretations of quality (3 and 4) exhibit the problems which afflict the rest of the genus. But with these examples it is also interesting to note the explicit attempt to harmonise 'best' and 'cheapest'. NHS policy-makers have long been aware that a genuine reconciliation of the imperatives to produce 'best services' at 'least cost' (i.e. 'basic principles' 3 and 4) is elusive (to say the least), so it is no surprise that this form of industrial camouflage has found favour. The contradictory principles appear to join under the banner of quality. At a stroke the impossible is apparently conceivable: top quality, satisfied customers, and at lowest possible cost.

Of course it is all a sham. Health care managers know very well that the best houses in their neighbourhood are not the cheapest. But in a bureaucracy where conformity overshadows reason to the extent that even obvious nonsense is immune from criticism (as demonstrated by countless contemporary health service documents), it has become possible for some to believe that the best really can be had cheaply.

5. Fitness for use or purpose.[57]

The most widely used 'definition of quality' – or at least definition of a 'quality product or service' – holds that 'if the product is fit for the intended purpose then it is quality' (the 'fit for the purpose' definition for short). The stress on purpose is encouraging (since deep consideration of the question 'what is the health service for?' is ultimately the only way truly to reform irrational NHS planning), but unfortunately this definition has the customary range of biases. These generate several problems.

By far the most significant of these is that this account does not require any stipulation of the 'purpose' that the service is said to be fit for. Consequently there is no condition set that 'the purpose' itself should be a quality purpose, or indeed any particular type of purpose. All that is required is that the object should be fit for some unspecified purpose. This lack of precision may be appropriate to business use where the primary concern is well known, but without an appropriate statement of purpose the notion is quite out of place in a health care system looking for a meaningful direction.

What works for a profit-making organisation with a clear primary goal does not work for an organisation where ultimate purpose is obscure, intensely debated, and rich in variety. The systems are worlds apart. Thus, the unreflective importation of business language into health care structures carries with it the implications that:

1. The nature of the overall purpose is irrelevant to judgements about the quality of the product or service. In other words, on this definition, it simply does not matter what the purpose is so long as there is some purpose that the service can be said to be fit for, and,
2. Judgements about what counts as 'quality in health care' can be made only by reference to existing purposes (since there must be some purpose to permit a judgement about quality). Therefore, in the context of the NHS the 'fit for the purpose' definition acts to set the level of quality in accord with whatever functioning service is on offer (since 'what is on offer' in the health service more than anything else, and certainly more than any plan, delineates its purpose). This implication fits perfectly with the three official health service definitions of need discussed previously. Far from being innovations in health service management, taken together they form a powerful defence against democratic reform.

All of which leads to the conclusion that the use of 'commercial definitions of quality' in the health service is not just inappropriate but, when taken out of a business setting, many of them can actually work to make health care more philosophically aimless. In business basic purpose is known, in health care it is not. In the absence of proper vision the only guide is what politics and the market happens to have put in place. This fickle master – not ideas, and not thoughtful blueprints – has come to be in charge of the NHS.

The Flight from Commonsense

Understood under any of the commercial options quality is not intrinsic to a thing. Yet in everyday life the opposite is true. A thing or person or event either is quality or it is not. Its status does not normally change according to variations in external circumstances. In commonsense something is either quality or not, full stop. The commonplace view tends to equate quality much more with 'excellence' than with what is valued at a particular time or place, or with what works. In normal circumstances if a person is asked to say what counts as quality in a familiar subject area it is likely that she will describe examples of very good practice, something above average, something worth writing home about. It is unlikely that she will point to anything unremarkable. For the lay person, quality is notable in some way.

If quality is taken to be dependent upon such variables as 'customer tolerance', 'meeting the needs of the market' or 'fitness for purpose' then it is necessarily defined relatively, and so must vary according to the task set (a phenomenon redolent of the 'general relativity' of health care purpose, pp. 9–10). The small lawn mower which is a quality mower so long as it cuts the customer's small patch of grass is not a quality mower if it is called upon to cut the grass in the local park. Since it is not up to this task it cannot be described as a quality mower. So simultaneously it can be both a quality and a non-quality object, however well or poorly made, and however technically advanced it is in its own right.

But this is a very strange position, in which it is not the thing itself which is quality. Instead virtually everything depends upon the circumstances in which the item finds itself. Extending this logic, if – by some unlikely disaster – all the footballers in England were to be incapacitated apart from 10 players and myself, then I could play for England as a quality player since I would (just about) be 'fit for the purpose' of making the numbers up. But, as anyone who has witnessed my increasingly desperate efforts to play football will know, this is quite absurd. It is fair to say that I am not, nor could I ever be under any stretch of the imagination or even corruption of language – a quality footballer.

PART TWO

A Philosophical Understanding of Quality: or an Account from Outside the NHS Sub-culture

Clearly the use of the term 'quality' in health care has become considerably distorted from its 'ordinary usage'. Therefore, in order to establish a realistic understanding of quality it is necessary to take a few steps back, and to begin an assessment from basics.

Quality as an 'Approval Word'

It is common knowledge that the word quality is used loosely in daily affairs. Mr Kipling boast of their 'quality cake', MFI reckon to manufacture 'quality furniture', British Polytechnics (now 'new Universities') claim to supply 'quality teaching' (whilst at the same time admitting implausibly large numbers of students). Not infrequently the word 'quality' is employed merely to emphasise a preference, adding no substance beyond rhetorical appeal.

From Approval to Substance

The question is, does any means exist to judge whether the cake, furniture or Polytechnic teaching is truly of quality? Is there a purely objective method to decide, can quality mean anything anybody wants it to mean, or is there a middle road?

In order to see the way to an answer it is first necessary to identify those features essential to any judgement about the quality of something.

Prerequisites for Judgements of Quality

Prerequisite One: There Must be Standards

If quality is to be assessed it is necessary to have some standard against which to measure it. Quality does not exist absolutely, or independent of things and judgements about them, but is a relative term which depends for its meaning upon the possibility of other things or processes not being describable as quality.

If everything is described as quality the notion becomes meaningless, but not anything can count as quality (the 'comedian' who never makes anyone laugh, the writer who can never make his plot hang together – these do not exhibit quality because their purpose is not achieved). There are, in reality, limits on 'quality assessment'. It can be said that if something is **not** fit for its purpose it cannot be of quality since a basic standard of performance is not met. However, it does not follow from this that anything which is fit for a purpose is necessarily quality since the standard may be set higher than this.

In practice there may be a great number of questions to be answered about how standards ought to be set, and about who should set them, but the basic point to notice is that, whatever their source, there must at least be some standards to enable 'quality assessment' at all. The point at which this standard occurs may be given the label 'quality threshold'.

Prerequisite Two: Purpose Must be Understood

In order to set any standards at all it is necessary to have an understanding of the purpose of the thing or process in question, and in every case the specification of purpose must precede the setting of standards.

It is possible to set standards in various ways. The standard of something may be determined by its use, it may be set by a decision ('above this standard this is a work of art', for instance), and it may also be decided by reference to a broader context. The two former methods need not consider the more general effects of a thing. If something is up to historical or technical standards this does not necessarily mean that it is up to a standard where the broader purpose of the enterprise is taken into account.

To take an example from beyond the margins of health care, it may be that certain processes of torture can be admired for ingenuity, or that a torturer's thoroughness is thought exceptional. She may be able to torture with exquisite cruelty, and may produce quality in many specific aspects of her work. But only to assess the technicalities of torture – in the absence of a view on the overall purpose of the activity – is surely to make an incomplete judgement.

Prerequisite Three: In Order to Assess the Quality of Complex Services Thoroughly it is Necessary to Identify Specific Aspects

If quality is to be judged across the whole range of health service activity assessments must include as many **specific aspects** of health services as possible. Any complex product or service will have a great many aspects, some of these will be obvious and clear (for instance, the number of patients checked into a hospital ward each week) and some will be hard to explain and impossible to quantify (for instance, the fluctuating anxieties and moods of the patients as they are admitted). In order to obtain a balanced impression of the universal quality of an organisation it will be necessary to assess a representative range of specific aspects. There is an imbalance in current 'quality assessments', for the following reasons:

1. In current measurements of NHS 'efficiency' there is strong emphasis on 'output and outcome'. Despite some wishful thinking that 'outcome measures' should incorporate all possible benefits of health care, in practice this emphasis means that judgements about processes as a whole depend far more on the end results (or the final 'specific aspect') than on what happens during them (so a 'successful outcome' of a patient's hospital stay is much more likely to be thought of as the speed between entry and discharge – the 'time-span outcome' – and the success of therapy on the clinical condition, rather than the sum of experiences of the individual patient).

   If quality is not seen 'generally' but only in accord with one or two specific isolated purposes or end results, then a great deal else about the health care process is inevitably ignored. If a service is said to be not fit for a very limited range of selected specific purposes, then regardless of how good, or useful, or appealing, or enabling it is more generally, these features will be ignored in 'quality assessment' exercises. In this way the football team at the bottom of the league will, inevitably, not be of quality if their specific purpose is to become champions. It will not matter that they are fun to watch, if they produce exciting matches, if their passing skills are superb, or if their determination is admirable. If they are not winners, and this is the aspect that counts, they will not be quality. Equally, the potential medical student with all-round human skills and intelligence – but with only average grades in A-level sciences – is, in many medical schools, very unlikely to be assessed as a 'quality entrant'.
2. Those 'outcomes' or 'specific aspects' considered to be important are defined by those services which happen to be funded and in place since these are thought of as 'hard or factual aspects'. Such 'hardness' is commonly believed to override other considerations.
3. The 'outcomes' or 'aspects' which are currently assessed for quality are those which can most easily be measured – those which are most accessible to statistical analysis, those which are most readily countable.

As it is normally conceived quality is not thought to be something which can be known only by means of quantitative measurement. Indeed the opposite is more often true. However, in the NHS at the moment only a very small number of particular aspects of the health service are actually specified, measured and so assessed for quality. In fact, it is technically possible to measure only a tiny proportion of the full range of NHS activities by current methods. And where the spotlight falls on only a small part of the stage everything else must remain unseen.

What is more, even the most apparently simply quantifiable aspects of the service can be assessed in different ways, and by different methods. For example, numbers of immunised children can be counted and translated into percentages of the 'target population'. But, for exactly the same numbers, an assessment might also be made of the level of comprehension of each of the adults who gave the consent. Equally the quality of the administration of the injection can be assessed in accord with 'accuracy of injection site' (which may be measured on a calibrated scale), but the quality of the injection might also be judged in accord with the level of anxiety of the recipient, and its after-effects on his behaviour. In part these alternatives are not entertained because they are more difficult to do, but the imbalance is also a product of a wider cultural malaise in which only those outcomes which can be 'objectively witnessed', and only the most indisputable findings, are thought to be important.[58] In this atmosphere, rather than seize on disputes as opportunities for innovation and improvement; controversy, variety and disagreement is thought of as signifying instability – apparently a problem to be avoided at virtually any cost.

Health Care Process as Successive Mini-purposes

One way to counteract this trend is to think of every process as a succession of mini-purposes in which every aspect is as important as any other. That is, to think of every part of health care activity as something which might be assessed for quality or not. In this way a much richer appreciation of the quality of activities is guaranteed. Think of the complexity of the nursing involved in terminal care. The final outcome is almost always the same at the end of each complicated process – a dead body to be dealt with and a bed to be stripped down. But of course it is not this result or aspect which counts – it is everything else that takes place as part of the process (or, all the other results or aspects which together make up 'the process leading up to the end result'). To separate the 'final aspect' or outcome from other aspects is a quite arbitrary thing to do. All aspects have their place. The nurse's emotions, what the nurse says, how the nurse deals with relatives, what the nurse thinks, how the nurse perceives the person, how the person perceives the nurse, each technical procedure – all of these things constitute health care activity. If the quality of the nurse's work is truly to be assessed then a 'judgement of quality' should be applied to every part of the process. As a further example it may be that a surgeon is consistently superb at achieving his ultimate end or purpose, yet regularly performs surgery on parts of the body he thinks necessary but to which patients have not consented. In order to consider the quality of his work in any extensive way it is not enough just to look at the ultimate 'successful outcome' – that is, that aspect where the clinical purpose of the operation is achieved. The operation must be examined in all its aspects if a complete judgement is to be made.

Prerequisite Four: Knowledge and Experience

Unless a person has **knowledge** and **experience** of a thing or process, she cannot possibly judge whether or not it is a thing or process of quality. This may seem an obvious point, but it is frequently ignored, particularly by those who believe that judgements of quality must be 'management led'. Consequently it is crucial to establish this as an axiom. A great deal rests on it if the NHS is to be opened up to public inspection and participation.

The Most Basic 'Quality Judgements'

Vegetables

Imagine that you are on holiday (or perhaps have recently taken a job in a foreign country) and someone asks your opinion of the quality of a vegetable which you have never seen before. You are told the vegetable is a **taro** but this means nothing to you. It is set out on a table with several other vegetables of the same type, and you are able to see that the variety can be of varying size and shade of colour. However, in your ignorance of taros the best you can do is hazard a guess based upon your general knowledge of vegetables.

Clearly you are in no position to assess the quality of the vegetable accurately, since you have no idea what the relevant standard is. From your general knowledge of vegetables you know that they should taste palatable – usually savoury, but not always – and that they should be nourishing – but not always. You know what vegetables are usually for, but you do not know about this vegetable. You do not even know whether it is best eaten raw or cooked. It is only after eating several, in various forms, that you become able to make any sort of judgement. And it may well be a considerable time before you can truly spot the quality vegetable.

Chairs

You are now in a room which contains six chairs, each a different type. Some are ornate, some plain, some comfy – but all can be sat on. Unlike the case of the vegetable, you have been given some guidance to enable you to make an 'informed judgement'. This time you know one 'rule of quality'. You know that if a chair can be sat on then it is a 'quality chair' – in other words you know that 'sitability' is one criterion of quality. Above this standard all chairs qualify as quality chairs. (Thus your rule is roughly the commercial rule – if it works and someone is likely to use it, then it is quality. And thus when you study the row of chairs armed with your regulation you are experiencing something akin to the thought process of a typical NHS manager.)

More Chairs

You are now in another room, with six more chairs. This time they appear identical. You are again asked which of them are 'quality chairs'. Of course you are getting wise to this now, and reply that either they are all quality or they are not, since they are identical. If 'sitability' is still the standard (or quality threshold) in this room then – since they can all be sat on – they must all be quality chairs.

However, you are not alone. Someone else in the room is also making a judgement. This judge happens to be a French polisher, and can see that one chair is polished to a higher standard than the others. In his view either they are as you say (if 'sitability' is the specified aspect) or, if the 'level of polish' is the specific aspect and the five adequately polished chairs set the standard for quality (i.e. they are the norm above which quality begins) then the well-polished chair is the quality chair. Alternatively, if the five adequately polished chairs are above a 'double specific' standard, and so count as quality for both 'polish' and 'sitability', then every chair is a quality chair on both counts. The only thing is, one is better than the others even though they are all quality chairs.

One by one further experts are introduced – one is an authority in aesthetics, another in carpentry, another in osteopathy and posture, another in upholstery, and so on until there is some considerable dispute about which are quality chairs, which are not, and which are the highest quality chairs. All of which confirms that judgements of quality – if they are to be at all penetrating – must take account of a variety of aspects of whatever is being judged. The judgements may be permanently controversial, and certainly go beyond whether some people are prepared to enter into a commercial transaction (people are very often acutely aware that the very last thing they are doing when shopping is 'buying quality'). If it is wished to avoid debate then the alternative is to select a few specific aspects, each of which can be fully assessed by the 'experts'. But, if a broad and comprehensive judgement is sought then much more flexible notions of quality are necessary – even for judgements about simple things like vegetables and chairs.

Levels of Judgement

There are different levels at which judgements of quality may or may not be made:

1. With no knowledge of any aspects of the thing in question, or with no specific expertise. In this case no meaningful judgement of quality will be possible.

2. Judgements of the most easily measurable, or most obvious, or most crude 'specific aspects'. In such a case a meaningful, but limited, judgement of quality is possible.
3. Complex judgements of quality which take account of as many different aspects of the thing in question is possible.

Most health service managers operate at levels 1 and 2 but hardly ever – if at all – at level 3. The effect of this is to restrict 'quality assessment' to a very limited number of aspects of the health service. This approach is normative (see pp. 30–31), and apparently safe from a requirement to involve others (that is to invoke level 3 correctly). This third level, which must involve disagreement, conflict, change, uncertainty and innovation is essentially democratic rather than normative.

Some Conclusions

A number of clear points have emerged from the foregoing analysis and examples:

1. *General and specific judgements.*
   Ascriptions of quality either can be made generally (and therefore vaguely – as in 'Fred is a quality person'), or can be made in relation to selected specific aspects (as in 'Fred's expertise in differential calculus is of high quality').

2. *Standards are necessary.*
   Whenever an aspect is being judged it must be assessed against some standard, whether this standard is made explicit or not. To assess quality in the absence of a standard makes no sense. (For democratic purposes standards must be made explicit and public.)

3. *The quality threshold cannot be set anywhere.*
   The level at which the standard is set (the quality threshold) can vary but cannot be set at just any level without rendering the notion of quality empty and meaningless.

4. *Deep disagreement is possible, but not necessarily undesirable.*
   Not only is it possible for people to disagree in their judgements about whether the same aspects are quality or not, but it is also possible for there to be disagreement about which aspect or aspects should be selected for judgement, and which aspects are more or less significant. However, if a rich view of the quality of something is sought then disharmony is a price worth paying.

5. *Different aspects will require different forms of assessment.*
   Given that most health service processes are complex and are made up of different aspects, different forms of assessment may well be necessary to assess the same process. For example, the assessment for quality of the number of operations performed by a surgeon (compared with the rate of

other surgeons) is of a different nature from the assessment of the post-operative well-being of patients. The latter is more difficult, and involves more complex considerations, but is not impossible in principle. The more difficult something is to do the harder it is to achieve, but increased difficulty does not mean increased impossibility. If it's possible, it's possible.

6. *There is no reason in principle why all aspects should not be assessed – size and complexity means more aspects and therefore requires more effort, but does not of itself rule out multifaceted assessment.*
   Anything other than the most simple of objects may have a number of purposes and will have many aspects. An organisation as large as the NHS is made up of an incalculable number of aspects. So long as specific quality thresholds have been set (and these will have many different natures in an organisation as large as the NHS) each of these aspects might be said to be quality or not. And with a little more sophistication, if degrees of quality are allowed, then each aspect may be said to be of 'good quality' or 'exceptional quality', and so on.

7. *To facilitate assessment it may be helpful to categorise processes in 'quality units'.*
   For convenience it may be helpful to amalgamate a number of specific aspects for assessment as a 'quality unit' (for example, a unit might be a ward, a doctor, a technical process, the effects of medication, or a committee meeting – each might be defined as a 'unit for assessment'). It may be a matter of convention which combination of aspects is said to make up a 'quality unit', or it may be to do with power and influence, but once 'the unit' has been established (in whatever way) it then becomes possible to assess the quality of that particular whole. The assessment will depend upon such features as where the standard has been set for each individual aspect of the overall unit, how each aspect is 'weighted' comparatively, and which aspects of the multitude of possibilities are selected for assessment at all.

8. *More knowledge generally means more profound judgements of quality.*
   Richer understanding of the quality of something composed of several aspects will grow in proportion to the knowledge and experience of the judge.

How might these points affect the NHS? If the idea of quality is taken seriously then:

> The fullest assessment of quality can come about only when the fullest account has been taken of the sum total of the specifics.

The quality of an organisation can be fully assessed only by reviewing every aspect of that organisation's work. There can be no doubt about this. In the NHS, as in commerce, there is a natural tendency to assess only those things which are easiest to assess to see if they exceed the quality threshold, but this is bound to give an unbalanced, misleading view of the activities of the organisation. For instance, staff/patient ratios can easily be calculated whereas staff morale cannot. But it is essential to assess both – in addition to an indefinite number of other aspects – if a thorough impression of the quality of health services is to be had.

The systematic measurement of diseases cured, operations done, or smears performed, will be necessary in a health service governed by a limited form of purpose (say, the efficient management of disease). But if this is the predominant type of 'quality assessment' done in a multi-purpose set-up (and it is undeniably prominent within the NHS) then this is unacceptable. Only if the NHS were truly a simple 'purposive' organisation in the way that a business is would such naivety be appropriate. And it is acknowledged, even by the most ardent advocates of TQM, that the NHS is more complex than this. For example:

> The imperatives to undertake TQM in the commercial sector are usually clear – to improve market share . . .

whereas the goal in the NHS is said to be to

> . . . improve the quality of care . . ..[50]

However, once this concession has been made others must follow. It is inescapably true that the whole **idea of care** is complex (contradictory in parts), and not simple, quite unlike the basic commercial aim. And once this is accepted it is easy to see how superficial the present notion of 'quality assessment' is.

The Relationship between Quality and Democracy

If quality in the NHS is to be comprehensively assessed then standards have to be set for each aspect of the organisation's operation. And since it is necessary to have a reasonable level of experience to judge quality (as can be seen from the case of the taro and the chairs on pp. 55–56), it is necessary to have the most expert people in each aspect of the service's operation to set the quality threshold for that aspect. In other words, everybody in the organisation must be involved if a proper 'quality assessment' is to be had: doctors, nurses, patients, technicians, administrators, secretaries, porters, managers – whoever happens to be expert and involved in whatever area of operation must have a say in what counts as quality, and what falls below the quality threshold. Without this it is inevitable that only a few standards will be set in relation to only a few aspects of the service's work. In this way the notion of quality can be used as one means to democratise the organisation. And this, after all, is one of the avowed intentions of the 'business gurus' who have so 'inspired' thinking about quality in the health service. Their aim too is to foster a 'quality culture' in which everyone is encouraged to have a say in the 'production process'.

It should be noted that I have made no mention in this paper of any definition of quality which I would wish to defend. In fact, quality is not so tangible that it can be precisely defined. However, if quality is to be taken as a serious idea in the NHS then certain requirements are necessary. And further, if these are taken seriously then certain other conclusions for the design and operation of a health service must surely follow (see pp. 121–128 where I outline the framework for my preferred option).

Paper Four

Equality

PART ONE

Equality in Health Care – the Ambiguous Principle

In 1948 Aneurin Bevan affirmed that one of the purposes of the NHS was 'to provide the people of Great Britain, no matter where they may be, with the same level of service'.[59] His apparent intent was to apply a socialist principle to remedy an 'obviously unjust' situation in which people received better health care if they happened to live in well-resourced areas, or if they were rich enough to afford private medicine.[60]

Ever since, the belief that 'the health service should be for all the British people equally' has been a deeply cherished – yet generally unexamined – NHS principle.[61] For many it appears morally indisputable that everyone – whatever their nature, whatever their circumstances – should be equally entitled to state funded health care. Thus, Bevan's explicit assertion of the principle of 'equality in health care' is commonly thought to be nothing more than the proper acknowledgement of a generally accepted 'moral right'. However, espoused in its most elementary fashion – as it is by countless defenders of the present NHS – theoretically it is by no means clear why equality is such a good thing, nor is it easy to see how the principle translates into realistic work practices.

In essence Bevan's 'equality principle' states that everyone should have the same chance to gain access to whatever medical services are available at a particular time. This view is sometimes converted into the assertion that there should be 'equal access to health care', and sometimes into the statements 'equal access for equal need' or 'equal access according to need'. These expressions are not entirely synonymous, but do share the characteristic that none of them can be systematically applied after philosophical analysis without causing considerable theoretical and practical controversy.

The fact that it is unusual to encounter any fuss over the 'equality principle' does not mean that it is clear and accepted. On the contrary, the lack of debate is merely evidence that few in the health service ever try to use it seriously. Thus, contrary to the fashionable belief that equality at least is an unequivocal NHS principle, this paper argues that the NHS does not have a coherent egalitarian philosophy, and so possesses no practical egalitarian impulse to guide planning.

In fact the aspiration to 'equality in the health service' could hardly be more vague.[62] However, as the emphasis on rationing, 'health care markets', and allocating resources in line with 'personal behaviour' grows increasingly strong, philosophical ambiguity over the meaning of equality can no longer be overlooked. In the absence of detailed analysis the principle of equality is in danger of disappearing altogether as a substantial idea in health care. If egalitarianism is to stand for anything in the NHS, and certainly if egalitarian policies are to be enacted, then the question **'what should equality in health care mean?'** must now be faced.

It is not always easy to see what is problematic about this question since the matter seems superficially so simple – equality must mean equal benefits for all. But this is not the only possible meaning of equality in health care. There is more than one way of understanding the idea, and so alternative practical policies which the notion of equality in health care might inspire.

The most elementary oversight sometimes made in assertions about equality in health is the assumption that the same for everyone means a decent amount for everyone. But taken in its purest sense 'equal shares for all' need not have this implication. Certainly 'the same level of service' may mean 'the very maximum level of service on every occasion'. For instance, 'health' could be made the topmost national priority, and money spent on other social provision only once the NHS is saturated with sufficient funding to guarantee everyone whatever medical service is required. However, it is also quite possible for the phrase 'the same level of service' to mean that everyone should get nothing. So, far from being a 'moral certainty', Bevan's aspiration to equality begs the daunting practical question: 'What level of medical provision – if any – ought to be made available to everyone?'.

Geometrical Equality

'Equal shares for all' is essentially the demand that whatever the dimensions of the pie everyone should get the same size slice. Interpreted like this the notion of equality can have utopian appeal since it combines the simplest arithmetic with the most rudimentary morality to assert that all human beings are essentially equal. Its practical implication is that all people should enjoy similar benefits, and carry similar burdens in life. For instance, it might be argued under this view that all should receive identical wages, or should have a similar area of living space, or should receive the same medical care.

Such an understanding of equality has, for the past 50 years, underpinned part of the British welfare system. Over this period, through deductions in their wages paid to a National Insurance scheme, British citizens have earned the right to state pensions and child benefit. Above a 'low ceiling' the deductions have been the same no matter what the level of each person's salary, and to date all citizens remain equally entitled to Child Benefit and various pensions, whatever their general circumstances.

The Difficulty of Geometrical Equality

Once the theory and practice of this – or any other – policy of 'equal shares for all come what may' is examined, serious weaknesses become apparent. The simplest example is sufficient to demonstrate the problem.

Equal Shares are not Necessarily Fair Shares

An academic department is proud of its 'egalitarian policies', which it interprets geometrically. It is a 'clinical department' with two main functions – teaching and research within its own medical speciality. The department houses two 'non-clinical' academics, and six clinicians. Within this department, as within any department in a university medical school, there are two salary scales – one for the clinicians and one for the non-clinicians. The clinical scale pays at a significantly higher rate across all categories than the non-clinical one.

Each year the department receives a concession from a central fund to help pay for academics to attend conferences. The concession is not large but can defray the costs of a return fare to London. According to its 'egalitarian policy' the department splits the fund equally between each academic.

The basic difficulty over the fairness of such a policy is clear. Those in receipt of benefit from the fund are not, **in general**, in equal positions. Their circumstances can be considered equal only if they are viewed in an **artificial** fashion. The academics can be thought of as equal only if **every factor of difference is ignored.** Before a policy of geometrical equality can be applied it is first necessary to constrain or define the situation and people in question by means of a human judgement about what is and is not relevant. In the case of the academics, considerations such as contrasts in personal income, and in need to attend conferences (in which category there may be many variables including frequency of past attendance, the need to present research findings to peers for discussion, and the need for academic stimulation) must be disregarded. A policy of geometrical equality can seem fair only if what is allowed as relevant to the situation is kept within very tight limits. Frequently, as in the above example, one factor only is said to be relevant (in this case everyone is an academic and therefore taken to be equal).

Where people's circumstances and desires are inextricably and complexly connected, a policy of geometrical equality can be successful only if people are happy to assume what is hardly if ever the case – that all people are equal in every truly relevant respect. In other words the policy can work only if each situation is converted into an **artefact**. Only if people are thought of in the most unrealistic fashion can it meaningfully be said to be egalitarian for a wealthy person, who can enjoy a high standard of living without a state pension, to be awarded one nonetheless. In the same way, if artificial models are disallowed, the claim that everyone should in principle and practice have a right to the same level of medical care is unsupportable. Once practical consider-ations are taken into account, to assert an actual right of equal access to medical services is mindless. Such a claim takes only the most limited account of people's real lives and circumstances, and so – sooner rather than later – is bound to result in injustice. It is obvious that people have different needs and so require different, not equal care. Not every group of people has equal need of cancer prevention work since cancers tend to proliferate more in some areas of the country, and in some sections of the population, than others.[40] And – obviously – only people with cancer have need of treatment. In such cases – and very clearly in the latter case – a policy of 'equal shares for all' is not practically persuasive. Instead a policy where those in the worst positions are given benefits first (sometimes called 'positive discrimination') seems intuitively much more fair. 'Equal shares for all regardless of circumstances' is 'blanket egalitarianism' – a universal policy which covers everyone in exactly the same way. But unless those underneath the blanket are all equal in the first place the strategy inevitably tends towards inequity (since people are not considered uniquely, and not treated in proportion to their circumstances).

Meeting Needs to 'Equalise'?

Because of the potential for injustice associated with planning in line with geometrical equality, to allow equal access to required resources only if there is equal need of them can be a more appealing alternative. Such a strategy may function to reduce and (at best) minimise the differences between people's circumstances, tending to **equalise** rather than treat them all in the same way. However, although this form of equality policy can act in a very different direction from the geometric version, it can be argued that this approach too does not consider people in proportion to their circumstances. For example, a common objection is that an equalising policy causes better off people to feel aggrieved if they believe they deserve to be better off as a result of their efforts in life (this is the classic 'American complaint' against the award of welfare benefits to those considered to be undeserving). Despite such protests, many egalitarians have argued that this strand of equality policy is the fairest.[63,64]

However, although a policy based on meeting need does take some account of people's circumstances, and is thus not so often obviously unjust as geometrical equality, its translation from abstract theory to complex practice is just as problematic. Unless only hypothetical examples or the most uncomplicated cases are considered, this form of egalitarianism is also artificial.

Which Needs Should Count Equally?

If it were the case that only a small range of health services were on offer – say it had become impossible for medicine to treat anything other than heart disease – then (if all possible heart disease treatments were fully available at no cost to other parts of society) it would be feasible to allow all heart disease sufferers equal access to 'heart services' in line with simple geometrical equality – everyone could have access without question. But if the full range of 'heart services' were not all available then uncomplicated equal access would not be possible. In such circumstances a policy of rationing based on need might be adopted instead. As has been seen, such a policy is described in various ways in the NHS. Sometimes it is said to be 'equal access for equal need', at other times it is cast as 'equal access according to need', or it may just be 'access according to need'. Each places need before equality as the governing factor in any deliberation, but only the latter expression makes no mention of equality. This version follows the full logic of the move to need and makes equality (or at least geometrical equality) irrelevant. It does not, however, undermine egalitarianism.

Applied to the example, those patients with equal needs would be guaranteed identical entry to services, and those with the greatest need would be attended to first. This would mean that a myocardial infarction would most probably be dealt with in preference to routine by-pass surgery, while two patients with mild angina would face a similar wait for attention. However, such a system of resource allocation appears realistic only if cast hypothetically, as simply as it is written above. In reality, where services are offered for a great range of conditions – in miscellaneous hospitals and health centres – and are designed to meet different types of need (physical, psychological and budgetary – to name but a few), enacting policy in line with the principle 'equal access according to equal need' is fraught with practical difficulty, and may be simply impossible to achieve if all germane variables are entered into the deliberation. Should Mr Smith in Carlisle have the same access as Mr Jones in Brighton? According to the clinicians he has equal need for medical treatment but, unlike Mr Jones, has no family. However, Mr Smith has the more active life, and so will probably do more as a result of the operation, will probably convalesce more quickly, and has a very strong will to go on living. Mrs Brown needs psychological, financial and family support to enable her to have the same operation as Mrs Green (who needs none of these props) – should she nevertheless have equal access to the medical service? Even at this fairly elementary level of complexity it seems impossible to apply the rule 'equal access according to need' – other than extremely superficially – even within single hospitals never mind across health authorities, since the wherewithal to balance even the most basic range of life variables is quite lacking in the health service at present.

'Pure Clinical Need' is also an Artefact

One obvious practical strategy is to offer access to medical services strictly in accordance with degree of clinical need (here defined simply as 'need as assessed by those with expertise in medicine'). But this option raises a similar conceptual problem to that found in the case of the academic allowances – it is possible to talk of clinical need as a **separate category** only with a great deal of philosophical juggling. Clinical need – just like the medical enterprise itself[65,66] – can rarely if ever in reality be separated off from non-clinical factors.

In most cases the very notion of clinical need actually **includes** such considerations as the 'general state of health' of the patient, the likelihood of success of the clinical intervention, and predictions of need for future medical therapy. Thus, although it might be true that there is a chance that a heart transplant in a 72-year-old person might be of benefit, and some doctors might even consider performing such an operation, it is not possible to say simply that there is therefore a clinical need for the transplant. Other factors simply must be taken into account, and these other factors (the person's age, whether she is robust, what facilities are available to her to help her convalesce, whether there are other potential recipients who might benefit more) are not directly clinical. The only way a pure notion of clinical need can be sustained is for any condition which might possibly be changed for the better through clinical intervention always to be defined as 'certainly needing medical help'. But if such a simplistic notion of clinical need were to be adopted 'clinical judgement' or indeed any form of intelligent discrimination would be ruled out. To say that a person 'needs medical help' is not a verdict which, in an adult world, ought to be arrived at merely through some form of technical test. Judgements of clinical need must, apart from the rarest of cases, involve broader deliberation (Is it worth the risk? How much will it cost? Does the patient want my help? How will the patient's working life be affected as a result of my clinical intervention?). If the rich and varied interconnections of the practical world are not artificially excluded no clinical problem is exactly identical (unless people with diseases and injuries are regarded as having no history, no identity, and no life outside the doctor's door).

PART TWO

Alternative Versions of Health Service Egalitarianism

Although in many circumstances a policy of 'equality in the health service' reduces logically to a strategy based solely on need (and then faces all the difficulties outlined in Paper Two), equality is still favoured by some as a basic – even the most basic – NHS principle. Arguably, it lay at the very heart of Bevan's reforms, even if political compromise meant that it could not be fully realised. However, if the principle is still to be taken seriously, a more substantial understanding of the notion is surely required.

In order to provide a positive account of equality in health care it is helpful to distinguish the alternative versions as clearly as possible.

Two Strategies: Blanket Equality, or an Equalising Approach?

Although it may look as if there are several equality options open (equal shares for all, equal access for equal need, access according to need) they can be distilled down to two essential forms – the **blanket** and **equalising** approaches. The latter category appears significantly different dependent upon whether the NHS is thought to offer 'medical services' or 'health services' – and this ultimately depends upon the way in which health care purpose is understood.

Blanket Equality

1. *Equality regardless*
   This strategy insists upon equal access to medical services for everyone, regardless of any other considerations.

Equalising

2a. *Equal help for equal 'clinical need' (or, help offered according to the severity of need as judged from the perspective of medicine).*
   This strategy urges that health service benefits should be distributed equally if people's clinical needs are identical, and unequally if these needs are not the same. Consequently, so far as clinical conditions are concerned, the strategy will tend to reduce differences between people since those with the severest diseases, injuries and pain should be treated as a priority if resources are limited and choices have to be made.

2b. *Help distributed according to health need perceived from a non-medical point of view.*
   This strategy offers health services (whether conceived solely as medical services or more broadly as welfare services of some kind) first to the most **generally** needy people. Unlike **2a** this strategy does not concentrate solely on clinical matters but takes at least some other life factors into account when deciding how to distribute benefits. Thus, under the interpretation where health services are thought of solely as medical services the strategy might, for instance, counsel that where private medicine is available, and where some people can afford to buy it and some cannot, state provision of health services should discriminate in favour of – or help first – those whose life circumstances do not equip them to pay for medical assistance. And under the interpretation where health services are conceived more broadly, if health services are thought to mean services beyond the clinical, and especially if they are interpreted as 'foundations for achievement'[67] then, by definition, they must be provided first to those with the most general health needs.

There are further variations on these themes. For instance, there is an option, governed primarily by a notion of clinical need but with account taken of some life circumstances, to treat the poorest people first where 'clinical need' is equal – and so use these people's more speedy 'return to health' as a **generally** equalising strategy.

Vagueness at the Outset

It is not clear which form of equality in health care was intended at the formation of the NHS. On the one hand the plan was said to be to 'provide all the people with the same level of service', but at the same time the idea was to establish 'a comprehensive national health service . . . (to) . . . ensure that for every citizen there is available whatever medical treatment he requires'.[68] Behind the apparently obvious fairness of these strategies lies a major confusion and a massive policy dilemma. To give everyone the same level of service seems to be blanket equality or **strategy 1**, and to offer medical services **as required** suggests access according to need or **strategy 2a**. What is more if it is true that illness/disease and health fall into quite different categories,[69] and such a view can quite reasonably be derived from the relevant government papers*, then the question is this: was/is the NHS meant simply to supply medical services to meet clinical needs (basically **strategy 2a**), and nothing more? Or was/is it meant to promote a much broader notion of health and well-being, where **strategy 2b** seems more appropriate? The way in which equality in health care is understood changes considerably according to which meaning is preferred – and each alternative has enormous implications for practice.

Four Assumptions

Historical research appears to show that the founders of the NHS interpreted equality in health care at times to mean blanket equality and at other times to mean the distribution of resources according to some form of assessed need. It is at least clear though that one intention of the 1946 emphasis on equality was to ensure that a person's geographical location did not affect his chances of receiving medical help, which it was thought ought to be the same wherever he happened to live. In other words, at least part of the inaugural aim certainly was to remedy a geometrical inequality produced largely by historical accident.

On the face of it this is a happy combination of both meanings of equality in health care (or at least of **strategy 1 and 2a**). However, this 'dual approach' can be said to be just or truly egalitarian only if certain very major assumptions are actually true. These assumptions are as follows:

Assumption One

That 'medical services' are a **special case.** Even if equal access for equal need is not possible for most good things in life (houses, boats and vintage wine, for instance) medical help is an exception. The belief is that medicine attends to **critical** problems, to matters of life and death – and thus that its concerns are of

---

* Note: The 1946 National Health Service Bill states: The Bill places a general duty upon the Minister of Health to promote a comprehensive health service for the improvement of the physical and mental health of the people of England and Wales, **and** for the prevention, diagnosis and treatment of illness (my emphasis).

It is enlightening to note the difference in meaning which would ensue if the penultimate 'and' in this quote were to be replaced by the phrase 'by means of' (deleting for).

a higher order to those of other agencies who devote themselves to the removal of other types of obstacle in life. It is, therefore, possible to distinguish the category of clinical need from other life needs (i.e. to invoke **strategy 2a**), and from general life circumstances. Medical priorities are simply special and distinct.

Assumption Two

That 'sickness' is 'no respecter of persons'. The assumption is, that unlike 'success in life' which more often than not depends upon the effort people are prepared to make, ill health is to do with chance or bad luck. In other words, disease might strike you down whoever you are, whatever you do and however you decide to live.

Assumption Three

(In keeping with assumptions one and two) 'medical services' are a special area of life, separate from wider social provision. Attention to health inequalities can therefore be carried out in a kind of vacuum. Since this is possible egalitarianism in the NHS can be enacted with a purity unattainable in other public enterprises. Consequently it can be said that in this area of human endeavour it is possible truly to treat people equally, without regard to class, gender, race or talent (i.e. to act in accord with **strategies 1 and 2a**). And that within the NHS it is possible to make interventions according to clinical need which will equalise people's (medically conceived) health status (i.e. **strategy 2a** where resources are limited).

Assumption Four

That because 'medical services' are special (assumption one), and because disease and illness can strike down rich and poor alike (assumption two), they should not be available only to those who can afford them or who live close to them, rather everyone should have access as of right (which is the Child Benefit and pensions argument in Britain).

In fact each of these assumptions is either false or contestable. Medicine is not obviously a special case, whether a person suffers disease or illness is not always only a matter of fortune, nor is it possible to treat clinical needs as an entirely separate category to other life needs. NHS egalitarianism cannot actually be carried out in 'splendid isolation', and it is not even clear and agreed that everyone should have access to medical services (some writers would exclude the poor and very old – see p. 118 – while others would bar the rich from state services).[70] Indeed, the pursuit of equality in health care can be counterproductive to the spirit of egalitarianism if sought in a social context which is not equalising in other significant ways.

Challenging the Assumptions

Of all the welfare initiatives taken half a century ago the National Health Service stirs the deepest feeling in the British people. It does so primarily because of a ubiquitous, usually unspoken belief that medicine is a unique enterprise, and a public medical service the only truly civilised response to the misery caused by sickness. These assumptions lie at the very core of the 'NHS myth'. However, they are not entirely true, and so cannot withstand open-minded analysis.

In order to gain a less biased understanding of equality in health care (and indeed to see the other NHS principles more clearly) it is essential to demonstrate that the assumptions cannot be sustained. Given the psychological inclination of most of the British public to believe in them (often with loud conviction and great passion) their refutation is far from easy. Proper thinking about health care is so often thwarted by a combination of false belief, indoctrination, authoritarianism, and media hype that it is difficult to see a way through to the truth. But the truth is there and, unwelcome as it may at first appear, is there to be understood.

Challenge to Assumption One

Are Medical Services a Special Case?

Consider the case of Wendy, as featured on the prime-time television series *Jimmys Watch*.

Scene One

The first time we meet Wendy she is not at all well. In fact we don't really meet her at all. Instead we see a trolley, complete with attendant drips, monitors and uniformed figures, being pushed along a hospital corridor with some urgency. The trolley supports a bundle of blankets and sheets out of which a number of tubes issue. With proper despatch the party disappears through two swing doors which, as all viewers know, can only lead to one place.

Scene Two

We still haven't met Wendy yet, although we do see a fair amount of blood and bile, and quite a bit of chopping and stitching.

Scene Three

At last we meet Wendy, sitting in her bed on the public ward. Although her situation is infinitely preferable in this scene, it is still far from ideal. Not only is she very hot from the television lights but she also has to answer vital questions which are being asked with the righteous fervour that only mass voyeurism can produce. 'That was a close thing wasn't it?', 'Do you realise how near you came to death back there?', 'Would you like to meet your parents now?'. It may well be quite a while before Wendy truly begins on the road to recovery.

Wendy's case seems to confirm the truth of the first assumption. She had to be admitted to the hospital for an emergency operation. If the skilled surgeon, the technology and the general hospital support had not been available then it is very likely that Wendy would have died. What then could be more obvious than the fact that Wendy had a critical problem of a nature quite unlike any other life problem she might encounter? In such circumstances does it not go without saying that her clinical need was quite distinct from her other needs, and entirely more important? Wendy needed a life-saving intervention, without which any more life (and so any further needs) would not exist. Her need was a clinical need, it was special, therefore medicine must be a special activity.

Refutation

So many legends have accumulated around the NHS that it seems nothing less than heresy to challenge the 'obvious truth' that what happened to Wendy belongs to a special category of intervention. But, even in such an apparently straightforward case, the first assumption can be shown to be fallacious.

It would be absurd to deny that Wendy faced a critical problem, and equally outrageous not to admit that her life was saved by the medical operation. However, this is not the assumption under challenge. What is contested is the belief that medical services – and even such acute medical services as this – are of a **different kind** from other types of service or help in life. On reflection it is clear that the difference in every case is a matter of **degree** and not a matter of **kind**. Sometimes there is no difference, in some cases medicine is the vital service, and in others non-medical services are most important.

Reflect upon what might have happened to Wendy had she not had her medical emergency. She was due to go on a sailing course at the weekend. If, during her tuition programme she had felt faint and fallen from her boat into the sea she would have been in a similar danger to that which she actually faced. Wendy cannot swim and, apart from her life-jacket (a literal life-support system), would be helpless in such circumstances. If her instructor had noticed her plight, and dived to her rescue (a move which, because of sharp rocks and fast currents, would have turned out to be difficult and technically complex) the situation would have paralleled the reality of her weekend in hospital. Wendy would have faced a critical, life-and-death problem, and she would have been saved by special techniques based on esoteric knowledge. The chances are that she might even have been interviewed afterwards.

Now, the question is would this rescue at sea – because of its unusual nature – have been of an entirely different order to other sorts of helpful maritime intervention, or would it only have been of a higher degree of seriousness than the norm? Put like this it is very clear that the rescue, however daring and complicated, does not fall into a special or unique category of thing, but is on a scale along with all other interventions to help people in trouble at sea. If Wendy had been out in a powerboat and her engine had failed – but she was not in any immediate danger – she would have required expert assistance to get her back to harbour. Wendy would still have needed to be rescued, and not everyone would have been expert enough to help her. The difference between this sea rescue and the first is simply that, in the latter case, there was not a life-and-death crisis. This shows two things which hardly need stating, but which are in effect denied by assumption one:

1. Life-and-death crises are not exclusive to medicine (indeed they are common to all emergency services and assistance).
2. Whatever the service, problems occur across a range of severity – from trivial to major.

It must also be pointed out that not all medicine deals with the sorts of emergencies which are so beloved of TV journalists with nothing to say. Much medical work is mundane and run of the mill. This means that conceptually there is no difference between Wendy going to her doctor for advice about the soreness in her left foot which is making repetitive use painful, and Wendy going to her jogging coach to see what his suggestions might be. Both experts will assess the problem from their different perspectives and advise according-ly. Indeed it is quite possible that both might recommend that Wendy goes to a physiotherapist.

It is important to remember that no need is necessarily absolute, nor is it in every case an imperative for a doctor or any other helper to act on even the most apparently compelling need (see p. 38). It is sometimes heard – from medical 'shroud-wavers' and other self-interested parties – that the difference between clinical need and other forms of need is that clinical need is somehow undeniable whereas other needs can be overridden. But this is not true. The clinical judgement of Wendy's surgeon about her clinical need is of the same type as the expert judgement of her rescuer at sea, and both might be overridden. For example, Wendy may be of a faith which will not accept the transfer of blood from one person to another, and this may be a fundamental belief for her. If so, her chosen instrumental need will act to override the normatively defined clinical need for the operation (and indeed any other instrumental needs of the doctor and the hospital which might also exist). Equally, Wendy's fall from the boat may not have been accidental. She may have jumped and may – for good reasons – wish to end her life in this fashion, in which case Wendy's most basic need will hardly be for a life-saving intervention.

However much blood is spilled, however many high-technology machines are invented, however impressive the discipline of medicine becomes it is not a special case, and so does not deserve special privileges drawn as if from some 'conceptual right'. Certainly medicine saves lives, but then so too do driving instructors, nurses, the police, housing agencies and employment exchanges. If a person has no job and a generally unfulfilled life he can 'die before his time' just as surely as he can if he has an internal haemorrhage and cannot get medical help quickly enough. And in those cases where life is not at risk the different agencies simply offer different varieties of help with life problems – the doctor may suggest anti-depressants for the unhappy man in a run down flat, the housing department may suggest a move, his friend may suggest a holiday, and the man may find his own solution in a new hobby. The medical advice does not fall into a different category of help – it merely lies in a particular field of expertise which has its own special interests and techniques. What is more, a great many medical services are in any case not developed by medicine at all, but by the massive industries of science and technology which direct their products at the medical market. If medicine is a singular case because of its special machinery then the industries which serve it must be more special still.

'It's not Medicine that's Special, it's Health!'

It might be argued that the real assumption is not that medical services are a special case, but that health is a special state: which is the inspiration behind such dubious proclamations as 'it does not matter too much if you are poor so long as you have your health', or 'I would give away all my fortune if I could only be healthy once more'. But this view is flawed too.[71]

Firstly, as noted in Paper One, the meaning of health is – as a matter of fact – given widely different interpretations, and so is thought to be very many different states. It is unlikely that so many ways of understanding health can all be special cases. Secondly, whatever health means – even if it is said to occur only in the absence of disease – it can be achieved in a range of ways, not just through medical interventions. And thirdly, it is not necessarily true that health is a value-free benefit which everyone desires equally. If, for instance, health is said to mean 'the absence of disease' then it is quite conceivable for people to 'trade off' a loss of health for other benefits – indeed this regularly happens. For example, people often work hard – or play hard – in the expectation that this might produce a medical problem. It may not be the case that these problems are actively sought, but if they are a known consequence of other activities and these activities are nonetheless still undertaken, then it is clear that health – at least health conceived in this crude way – is not the first priority (and certainly not thought of as a special sort of thing.)

Challenge to Assumption Two

If there is such a thing as luck in life then the second assumption is undeniably partly true. Some people hardly ever seem to be sick while others are plagued with illness and injury; some people can smoke, drink and party apparently without ill-effect while others can 'look after themselves' fastidiously and still become seriously ill. However, although most people can give examples of good and bad luck 'in health' the second assumption is far from being wholly true. Yet at the inauguration of the NHS it appears that this assumption was generally believed to be entirely correct. Seen 'through the spectacles of 1944'[72] fate does indeed seem to be the arbiter of sickness: just as a V2 bomb might have fallen on you wherever you happened to be in wartime Britain, so cancer or emphysema might strike at anybody, out of the blue. Since this was thought to be true, since in health at least higher social class and other privilege offered no protection against fortune, it was believed to be perfectly egalitarian to treat everybody as exactly equal in this regard. Health was thought to be a lottery which the civilised social planner would devise a system to beat.

Today this theory may still be true for some health problems although there are many, particularly those engaged in epidemiological work or in investigation within the social sciences, who would call into question the role of pure fate in any example advanced. On the face of it anyone who drives a car has the same chance of being injured on the roads through no fault of their own. But in fact it is not this simple. A driver's risk of being in an accident increases with the mileage covered, and also rises if alcohol has been consumed.[73] Risk of serious injury tends to depend on the size of the vehicle, and the extent of the manufacturer's safety precautions (which normally improve in proportion to the financial cost of the vehicle). Likewise, while it is true that any of us may suffer from cancer, and that in this very general sense we are all equal, it is now very well known that the chances of a person suffering cancer depend upon a range of variables which are not themselves simply dependent upon luck. For instance, a person's work, drinking and smoking habits, living conditions, level of stress, and even place of residence all affect the probability of developing cancers. In this sense we are not all equal, and may not in truth be equally susceptible to any medical problem.

These hard facts contradict the simple interpretation of equality in health care. The problem is this: if everyone is equally liable to contract medical troubles then medical services ought to be equally available to all people. If everyone is in the same boat then it is only fair that everyone should be treated alike. However, if it is not true that everyone is equally prone to medical troubles then – unless blanket equality is simply thought to be desirable whatever the surrounding inequalities – an egalitarian policy should attempt to compensate for the differences.

At present, whenever equal access or equality is advocated and defended as an essential part of the NHS, a quite artificial separation of 'medical' and 'life' circumstances is made. This separation has at least three psychological stages. First it must be believed that medical problems fall into a special category of problem, then that medical problems are largely or even entirely the result of misfortune whereas most other problems are not, and then that there must be a special service devoted exclusively to the solution of the special problems. Once one stage is accepted it is easy to accept the others, and when all three are held together they support each other in such a way that it can be very hard to shake one's thoughts loose of their shackles.

Challenge to Assumption Three

In many respects thinking and research about inequalities in health has progressed since the 1940s. Luck is now rarely discussed as a major factor in the incidence of disease, and differences in the way people are able to live are very often cited as crucial. However, such is the strength of the various NHS myths, that despite developments in the understanding of causes of 'ill health' a distinction is still regularly made (albeit often implicitly) between:

1. **'Health inequalities'** (which are generally considered a bad thing, and almost always said to be in need of reduction by improving the status of the 'most unhealthy'), and
2. **'Inequalities between people in general'** (which – unlike health inequalities – are not always said to be bad, and which are sometimes seen as either inevitable, desirable or both).[74]

The general view taken by those who maintain this distinction is that health care activity is, or certainly ought to be, work to reduce inequalities in people's health status (a notion which, like 'health benefit' and 'health gain', is – at best – vaguely defined in the NHS). However, it is rarely argued that the aim of health work is or ought to be to seek to reduce other inequalities between people. If it is, the strategy is always justified by pointing to anticipated improvements in health status. It may be that, as a **secondary consequence** of labour to improve this health status, some people's life circumstances improve. But this is seen more as a happy coincidence than a primary intention. There is, for instance, a tradition to improve 'public health' by the general provision of better sanitation, houses and nutritious food. And thus it is true to say that through its many projects to 'improve health' the 'public health movement' has often achieved social reform, but these activities are not usually undertaken because they are, in themselves, good things to do. In every case the pay-off of the work is thought to rest in better morbidity and mortality statistics (or at least this is always the publicised claim). These medically defined benefits are invariably seen as the proper justification for public health interventions, and typically are held to be uncontroversially good (or at least are said to be value-neutral, objective, or scientifically based – which amounts to the same thing for many observers).

Part of the reason for this emphasis on 'measurable health outcomes' is that it makes it much easier to tackle health problems without creating a debilitating political fuss. Although it is nowadays commonplace to resist increases in spending on public works, few politicians like to be seen to oppose improvements in health. However, the belief in the distinction between health inequalities and other inequalities is more deep-seated, and the source of its development much more profound, than can be explained by political expedience alone. Although some 'health campaigners' deliberately use health as a political shield there is much more to the perception that health and health services are a special area of life than this.

Consider an illustrative quote:

> The question is whether there is room for a direct shift of resources from curative to preventive medicine when there is little or no growth in the economy and little opportunity to increase the overall resources for the health service . . . (Douglas Black has explained) . . . we were all agreed that education and preventive measures, specifically directed towards the socially deprived, were necessary. But the sociological members of the group considered that the consequent expenditure should be obtained by diversion from the acute services. On the other hand the medical members felt that the acute services played a vital part in the prevention of chronic disability and could not be further cut back without serious effects on emergency care, on the training of doctors for both hospital work and for family practice and on the length of waiting lists.[75]

Although this discussion is focused on the problems of the generally 'socially deprived' it nevertheless appears to accept wholly the distinction between health inequalities and other inequalities. The problem is not seen as social deprivation itself (or at least this is not seen to be the appropriate problem to tackle), but what to do about the health problems social deprivation causes. Yet if it is the case that social deprivation causes diseases (as it clearly does)[75,76] then the obvious thing to do is not to increase 'education' and 'prevention' (however unequally or equitably targeted), but to do something about the deprivation in the first place. Of course this was not the province of the authors of the Black Report.[77] However, the principal reason it was not thought to be 'part of their agenda' was that an attack on social deprivation *per se* must involve addressing 'inequalities in wealth' or 'inequalities in people's opportunities to have a fulfilling life' (which are much more obviously sensitive topics). It is still very common to think that inequalities in health have more to do with biology than politics – that they are clinical rather than social matters. Thus – to take a very crude model – it is as if there are two boxes (see Fig. 5).

Within Box A symptoms are treated, whether or not they are caused within Box B. The argument of both factions of the Black Committee is to focus on the amount and distribution of resources within Box A in order to tackle these symptoms (a pattern which is exactly repeated with the use of the quality adjusted life year (QALY) in the health service – see Paper Five). In other words, under this assumption, it is felt to be correct to undertake health work in line with **strategy 1**, or **strategy 2a**, but not in keeping with **strategy 2b**.

B Existing social order and living conditions (creates those 'cases'
for system A which cannot be explained by ill fortune). As far as
health services are concerned these social circumstances are
bad either solely or primarily because of the **symptoms** dealt
with in A.

A Within this box money and other resources are moved
around in an established system. This system has not been
planned according to clearly worked out theories, but has
evolved and so has arbitrary boundaries. Within the system
priorities do change, but they do not always do so for
rational, argued reasons.

Fig. 5

Challenge to Assumption Four

If medical services are exceptional in the way they are popularly believed to be
(as follows from the first three assumptions), then there should be no
discrimination about who should and should not be able to use them. Everyone
should have equal access and/or access as required – in accord with the general
sentiment of 1946. However, since the other assumptions are not true then
neither is this one.

This may appear an outrageous thought, but it is not really so shocking.
Discrimination is already a fact of life in current health services – some sorts of
health services are as a matter of fact equally available to all (accident and
emergency services, for instance) but other types are only open to limited
groups (for instance, screening services and free prescriptions). And where
there is only so much money available to the system, when one group of people
gain, others are bound to lose. For example, money spent to ensure that all
people have equal access to general practitioners on the NHS (which they may
or may not need) means that money cannot be spent on providing nutritious
food (which could be explained as 'health promotion' for the purpose of being
'politically correct' within the NHS) as a right for all members of the
community.

Once more the problem reduces to the single, central fact that the health
service does not possess a set of coherent purposes. Of course, as this discussion
of assumptions shows, there are many other large conceptual problems facing
the NHS (most of which are never debated), but they all stem from the
confusion over health service purpose. The massive question which hangs over
the entire puzzle about who should get what stems directly from the heart of this

darkness: **according to what grand scheme are the winners and losers of this lottery decided?** At the moment, of course, the only answer is that there is no coherent scheme.

What Now?

If none of the four assumptions can be sustained, what are the implications? What alternatives are there?

In fact very many methods exist to enable the allocation of health service benefits, some of which are discussed in Paper Seven – Options and some of which are more moral than others. Prima facie, the following are of most striking relevance at this stage of the analysis. These are:

1. That access to medical services should remain 'blanket' as a matter of doctrine (**strategy 1**).
2. That 'core medical services', paid for through taxation, should be made available to all, and that beyond these services priorities should be set to 'filter' potential recipients of other services, so that the neediest receive help first (which should also be paid for out of taxation)[78] (**a combination of strategies 1 and 2a**).
3. That there should be 'core medical services' available to all paid for out of general taxation, but beyond this people should be left to buy what they want within their means (the American 'first and second class systems') (**a restricted version of strategy 1**).

(The above three options assume that medicine is special)

4. That since there is no special case for medical services these things should be supplied in just the same way as any other purchasable commodity. Since the uniqueness of medicine is a fiction the benefits of medicine should be distributed according to the market, just like all other benefits (cars, houses, holidays, etc. . . .) which it is felt appropriate to distribute between individuals in this way (**'equality' is an irrelevance according to this 'market option'**).
5. Rather than have 'core medical services' there should be 'core health services', by which a very different combination of benefits may be meant.

   On this view, if priorities for action have to be set, then it is not clinical need but a wider notion of health need which should inform the decision. If a choice has to be made between dealing with the dispensing of vitamins (for a person who needs them) and dealing with housing a person (where both things are possible) then the health question is not necessarily 'what is the clinical priority here?' but 'which alternative will have the most effect on increasing the general level of fulfilment of the person?' It may be that the answer is 'the vitamins' (maybe the person is not particularly disabled by living as an itinerant but is made very ill by vitamin deficiency) but it is more likely that the house should be provided first (**strategy 2b**).

The present system in the UK is a messy, incoherent compromise between options 1, 2 and 3. It cannot be justified philosophically and its proper reform has been delayed by a combination of mythology and self-interested, well-established power. Health services are supposed to be available to everyone equally, but in fact very many of them are not. It is true that the poorest (and youngest and oldest) people do not have to pay some or all of the direct NHS charges, but this is at best a most half-hearted attempt at 'equalising'. (A truly equalising policy would charge the most wealthy people the market rate for the service offered, and redistribute the profit to the direct advantage of the worst off people.) People are still filtered away from and towards services in very many ways (including discrimination on grounds of age, behaviour, class, geographical location, and services available). And, of course, if you have the money (or the insurance) you can buy whatever medical service the market can provide, within your means.

All the above are options for the 'definition of purpose' of the NHS. The first accepts that the 'four assumptions' are true while the others go against them to varying degrees. Options 4 and 5 (which will be discussed in more detail in Papers Six and Seven) are most obviously at odds with the four assumptions. Option 4 denies all four assumptions, and assumes that medicine is the same as any other service for sale, and that the same rules should apply as apply elsewhere in a capitalist society.

Option 5 also denies the four assumptions but takes a different line by retaining a belief in the worth of a more general equalising policy for health. The choice between these fundamentally different alternatives cannot be decided by recourse to a scientific test. Essentially these are different moral and semantic systems and so must be justified by other means.

Some Conclusions

The most central difficulty for the four assumptions and the combination of **Strategies 1** and **2a** is that health services do not take place in an ideal, hypothetical world, but in a world of enormous complexity. Even apparently minor decisions within health services can produce a profoundly complicated network of cause and effect. This can very often mean that an attempt at applying egalitarian policy in one respect acts to produce further inequalities in other, sometimes unexpected, areas.

Presently this truth is not taken into account, but instead it is passively assumed that blanket access and the provision of help according to clinical need is enough to ensure justice in medical services. But this can only be the case under the two following conditions, which in fact do not apply:

1. Apart from their clinical needs all people are otherwise equal.
2. Clinical needs are not caused by other inequalities external to the health care system.

The Illogic of Limited Egalitarianism

This is the central problem for egalitarians who urge 'health service egalitarian-ism' but do not – for whatever reason – extend their arguments beyond health care. It is an illogic with a number of causes, practical, political and theoretical, but which has in part resulted from a massive intellectual 'blind spot' in socialist planning.

The problem is that medical services (for this, for the great part, is what the NHS is) were singled out for special attention in the first part of the century, and especially in 1944–48. The reasons for this were that:

1. Medical services were very unevenly distributed, and this was 'obviously not fair'.
2. Sickness was debilitating, and a drain on the economy.
3. It was not felt appropriate that the wealthy should be able to afford the best medicine while the poor had to make do with what they could get.
4. Sickness was thought largely to be a question of chance – bad luck, not unequal circumstances.

Thus a 'comprehensive health service' open to all equally was proposed. However, despite the four reasons above there is no compelling reason why medical services should be a special case – it is equally possible to 'shroud-wave' in other areas of social provision. Thus there is no compelling reason why 'equal access for equal need' is exclusively appropriate to medical care. If the principle is so important then it should also apply to housing, transport, employment, higher education and so on. But it does not. And because it does not, because people's general needs are so unequal – to try to construct a specific 'egalitarian system' which is surrounded by non-egalitarian systems – cannot work.[79] Indeed, it will tend to promote inequality since the better off and better prepared tend to make better use of services.[80] Equal access to health services makes sense only if 'equal access for equal need' has first been applied to other areas of life so as truly to make illness/disease/sickness a matter of misfortune rather than something which could have been avoided given more general egalitarian planning.[81]

But this is not the place to argue this case in full. There is one more principle yet to be discussed which can offer a further insight into the philosophical health of the NHS.

Paper Five

Cost

PART ONE

Although there are some[82,83] who refuse to accept the view that 'health care resources' are truly scarce (arguing that any 'scarcity' is contrived, and that money could and should be diverted from 'defence' to 'health care', or should not be spent on 'luxuries' before 'health'), it is a matter of fact that the NHS has a limited budget provided by government and that not all of a nation's wealth can be spent on medical services. It also appears to be a universal rule that the fiscal costs of modern health services tend to rise, and particularly do so where the 'market' is allowed the freest hand in health care provision.[84,85] Where people wish to have the best services in order to be ever more healthy, where it is assumed that the most expensive services produce the healthiest outcomes, where there are considerable commercial incentives to market new technologies and drugs, and where the income of most types of 'health service unit' (defined on p. 58) is at least partly dependent upon attracting 'customers' in competition with other 'units', a quite devastating cocktail of self-interest exists. Unless rigorously controlled by the State this mix of desires combines to drain an ever higher proportion of a nation's resources. This pattern is now so well established and recognised as undesirable that limiting health service expenditure is a commonplace activity for the governments of most developed countries.[86]

In the US a range of tactics to control escalating costs is continually under consideration,[85,87] although many powerful commercial interests are determined to retain existing arrangements. In Britain, where the health service has traditionally been regarded as at least partly separate from the market economy, successive governments have nevertheless been constantly sensitive to the need to control the financial cost of medicine.[88] Prior to the mid-1980s costs were kept in check mainly through central control of the NHS budget. More recently (since 1984[89]), in keeping with the Tory government's long-standing attachment both to free markets and Victorian hierarchy, health service management was introduced to permit additional local control over costs. In 1990 this move was supplemented by the creation of 'internal markets' in the NHS.[90] Central government control of the health service budget is as tight as it ever was, but these extra measures give the appearance of government by delegation, and (in the minds of some people) have the added benefit of keeping everyone in the system firmly in their proper place, since virtually everyone is now accountable to his or her 'line-manager'.

However, despite the considerable political controversy generated by the influx of business talk and its associated techniques, these developments are nothing more than symptoms of the more central conceptual problems of the health service. Administrative changes make little difference to the overall balance of interests in the NHS. Accordingly, rather than dwell for long on whether or not 'business methods' are an appropriate means of 'cost-control' for a health service I propose instead to discuss the notion of cost *per se*.

Cost is an idea commonly used in health economics, where it forms part of a larger technical system. Following an exploration (albeit a very elementary one) of part of this system I shall conclude that a much clearer, more relevant and more basic interpretation of cost should be adopted. If this analysis of cost is accepted – and it follows quite logically from the general pattern of reasoning of health economics – then major implications must ensue. The way in which the identity of the NHS is understood, and the extent to which it is seen as an independent, special and autonomous organisation could be considerably altered as a result.

What is a Cost in Health Care?

Monetary Cost

At first sight the aim to keep health service costs to a minimum seems straightforward enough: it is as the governments of developed countries perceive it to be – a matter of spending money on health efficiently, and in reasonable proportion to spending elsewhere in society. Cost is very often popularly assumed simply to mean the financial price of something (as it is in the managers' budgetary reallocation dilemma), and indeed for many, cost-control in the NHS simply means the effort to maintain the health service budget below the rate of inflation. However, just as there are many different kinds of resource, so there are many different types of cost. Of course this is as true in business as it is in health care. But in health care 'human costs' assume a much greater importance than is usual in commerce, where success is ultimately judged on the evidence of financial balance sheets. Health services deal daily with pain, disability, birth and death. They constantly encounter many of life's most momentous events and so do not naturally reduce their actions and purposes to pounds or dollars. It is true that with effort almost anything in life can be assigned a monetary value, even the many and varied outcomes of health care. But such a crude translation of the results of health work is surely too limited.

Cost as Sacrifice

A less exclusive alternative to the above 'cash register view' is to define cost as the 'sacrifice' involved in the achievement of 'benefit'. Thus:

> To an economist 'what will it cost?' means 'what will have to be sacrificed?', and this may be very different from 'how much money will we have to part with?'. So if someone says to me

that they must have something **no matter what it costs,** I take them to mean that they must have it **no matter what sacrifices have to be made.**[91]

The above homily is directed against doctors who expect the 'clinical freedom' to take any steps they regard as necessary for the health of individual patients. The author believes that such a view is nothing more than 'fanaticism' since (in a system where resources are finite) whatever benefit is gained for one individual must sooner or later be had at the cost of a benefit which might otherwise have been enjoyed by someone else. Quite simply, the idea is that:

> In reality the cost of whatever you do with resources is the best of the other things that the resources could have been used for . . .[92]

The implication of understanding cost in this way is that in order truly to know what something will cost it is necessary to grasp fully the nature of the range of possible benefits which might be had (and therefore to know the degree of severity of all potential sacrifices). Now, if it were possible to interpret benefit as a simple unit (or 'utility') then the calculation of cost would not be especially difficult. If this were to be the case then health economists could, for instance, easily calculate the 'sacrifice cost' of a choice to offer a therapy to produce **three units of health benefit** for one patient instead of a therapy which would generate **10 units of health benefit** shared equally between five. In these circumstances cost would not be explained ultimately as money or time, but as the loss of the **seven units of health benefit** which might have been gained had the doctor been less of a fanatic.

If all this were so it would be logical to assume further that:

> (Efficiency in health services means) . . . concentrating resources on those effective services, provided at least cost, which offer the biggest pay off in terms of health.[92]

But in reality this statement can be usefully applied only if the nature of 'effective services' is both constant and clearly understood – as it would be if the services in question were carpet-cleaning or lawn-mowing – and only if 'the biggest pay off in terms of health' is truly determined (as it must be if 'least cost' is to have any meaning). An effective lawn-mowing service is readily specified and will most likely be understood in the same way by all customers and providers. If the mark of the successful or effective provision of health service X is taken to be the conceptual equivalent of a mowed lawn or a cleaned carpet, and if cost is conceived as money, then the mechanics seem appropriate. Understood in this way health service X can be said to be effective whenever outcome Y is achieved, and will be provided 'cost effectively' whenever Y occurs at the lowest financial cost. However, where the benefit or effectiveness of services is unclear, where costs are many and varied (as in real life), or where services have aspects which are weighted differently by people with different interests, such simplistic calculation is ruled out.

Health as the Profit of Health Care

A most basic and ostensibly reasonable assumption of health economists (and many of their detractors too)[82] is first that the 'profit' or benefit of health services is health, and second that health is a relatively unproblematic idea. If this were true then health economics would have a passable route from the ivory tower to health work reality. But whereas it is not difficult to understand that if Dennis buys a car on Tuesday for £100 and sells it on Wednesday for £120 (at the cost of a little time and a £5 advertisement) he will have made a financial gain, it is a much more complicated matter to judge the 'health profit margin' of health care interventions. In car-dealing the evidence of profit will probably take the form of three £5 notes, but (as earlier papers have demonstrated) in the case of health even what to look for as evidence of success or effectiveness will often be unclear. The crudest notions of health suggest that 'health profit' is simply and entirely indicated by reduced morbidity and mortality in populations, or disease cure and increased life expectancy in individuals. But these are only some of a wide variety of possible indicators of success.

Part of the problem is that while much recent philosophical research has begun to grapple with the complexity of the meaning of health this significant and serious academic problem is not yet of real concern to most health economists. Typically the matter is dismissed as if of very little importance. For example:

> I am going to assume, without much discussion, that the objective of health services is to promote health and, moreover, to do so in such a fashion as to maximise the impact on the nation's health of whatever resources are available to this end.[93]

However, in the absence of a realistic and practical understanding of health this brand of health economics is virtually metaphysical. It is left stranded as an abstract scheme in which only those meanings which suit the technical set-up are deemed germane. Whether the system makes sense as non-fiction is almost beside the point. Alan Williams admits as much:

> The difficulty about going beyond service **provision**, and examining instead service **benefits**, is that we have no **routine** data on the latter, and even research findings on the benefit of health care are patchy in both coverage and reliability . . ..[94]

Despite the lack of any conceptual or empirical justification 'service benefits' are nevertheless considered to be synonymous with health:

> I assume that benefits have been defined, measured and valued in a manner that is acceptable to everybody. In order to be as neutral as possible on that matter, I will, for expositional simplicity, assume that the health benefit we are talking about is simply one additional year of healthy life expectancy . . ..[94]

Now this is all very well if 'expositional simplicity' is what is required, but it is hardly an adequate means by which to understand and deal with **actual** problems of resource allocation. Indeed some of the assumptions of this version of health economics are so general (for example, that the 'objective of health services is to promote health') that strictly speaking they cannot be empirically refuted (although it is demonstrably incorrect to assume consensus on the definition of 'health service benefit'). However, they can all be shown to be simplistic, and so without doubt not a true representation of the reality of health services.

Proper Analysis of the Meaning of Health is Indispensable

It is worth re-emphasising this most central point. Health has multiple meanings and health work myriad shapes and numerous goals. Sometimes health can be understood in clinical terms, yet sometimes it makes no sense at all to interpret the word in this way. It is becoming increasingly widely acknowledged that health can quite properly mean more than the absence of a medical condition. Indeed, some health economists are now coming to recognise that the meaning of health must be analysed if their discipline is to progress any further.[95] In fact there are now several significant, philosophically argued theories of health in existence to which they might attend (see also pp. 10–11). These range from the view (1) that health should be understood as 'biological normality'[96] to an interpretation (2) of health as a person's ability to perform actions or reach goals in a social context.[97] Naturally these alternative accounts of health can suggest different practical directions for health work, and often imply very different interpretations of 'effective service', 'health pay-off' and 'health outcome'. For example, on understanding (1) 'effective-management' might require a painful or unwanted intervention to restore 'biological normality' while the second theory of health (2) might offer a conflicting notion of success, judging effectiveness ultimately according to the degree to which a person is able to live as she desires.[67] It may even be that a comparision of the costs of achieving such different yet legitimate health outcomes as **enabling a person to feel optimistic and full of hope for the future for a single day**, and **administering a course of childhood immunisations**, will simply not be possible because the benefits produced just do not fall within the same realm.[98] Indeed unless a meaningful common denominator can be found by which to appraise different health outcomes (or to understand 'the meaning of success' in the same way), attempting to assess multiple health benefits will remain the philosophical equivalent of trying to pass definitive judgement on the relative merits of a curry and a chrysanthemum.

Even if health economists and other health care policy-makers continue to ignore philosophical arguments, the fact remains that many diseases cannot be cured. As a consequence of this stubborn truth health services are – at this very moment – working to reduce pain or increase 'quality of life', sometimes even if this means not extending life expectancy and not working for 'biological normality'. Because these alternative ends actually exist the meanings of 'effective case management', 'health profit' and 'health care cost' are indisputably contentious, as a fact of life. Therefore, the cursory adoption of 'one additional year of healthy life expectancy' as a constant (yet obviously artificial) measure of outcome may not invalidate the internal logic of the economists' arguments, but it surely undermines any claim they may have to relevance.

Three Tactics to Ensure a 'Manageable System'

In order to keep the assessment of 'cost', 'benefit' and 'effectiveness' within reasonable bounds, health economists have developed three alternatives by which to control and mould the information they feed into their systems. Each of these tactics relies, in part, on accepting a parody of health service reality instead of working with reality itself. In this way the tactics share common ground with the attempts of some to carry out 'equality policies' within the NHS, in isolation from the more general application of such policies. The stratagems of the economists are:

1. *To take health to be an undefined 'good', about which discussion is barely necessary. On this strategy health economists are able to focus on provision rather than benefit.*
   This option simply assumes that whatever health services exist are provided for good reasons (and so inevitably produce health benefits). Since these good reasons and benefits are complex, and since the data on them are at best unreliable and at worst non-existent, the primary task of health economics is to work out the most efficient ways to provide current services.
2. *To take health to be the outcome of any effective clinical service, and to be quantifiable. The scope of this strategy includes analysis of health benefit, but only in so far as the notion is interpreted clinically.*
   On this strategy health is regarded as quantifiable (at least in principle if not yet always in practice). It is also assumed that health outcomes can be properly understood entirely within the framework of clinical practice. It is further understood that the health outcomes of different procedures will vary in degree of benefit. The research task under this approach is to identify the relevant clinical data as clearly as possible, and – by means of various health economic techniques – to analyse the levels of benefit produced.
3. *To designate health in such a way as to allow a more general quantitative/qualitative assessment of the degree of success of health care interventions. This technique takes a broader view of health and health benefit (although it tends to appear more narrow than it actually is).*
   This tactic eschews traditional clinical data, and instead makes use of 'the patient's view' of his or her 'quality of life' as part of the evaluation of health service outcomes. In so doing health benefits are assessed against cost in a way which goes beyond clinical outcome to encompass a more complete view of health. One ultimate aim of this strategy is to help assure the 'rational allocation of health service resources'.

PART TWO

The Quality Adjusted Life Year (QALY)

By far the most well-known instrument of this technique is the **QALY** or **Quality Adjusted Life Year**. The QALY has become a *bête noire* in various academic and health care circles, where it has been roundly criticised (usually with good reason) for such failings as ageism, sexism, preference for the fortunate, the 'false assumption' that health can be quantified, arbitrariness, cold utilitarianism, and the sabotage of clinical autonomy.[82,87] However, these criticisms are not the subject of this discussion, nor indeed are they the fundamental problem. In order to appreciate the essential weakness of the QALY it is necessary, and sufficient, to understand how the QALY was invented (it could never have been discovered). Briefly, the story is this.

The Invention of the QALY

The inventors of the QALY wished to devise a 'rough tariff' to represent the way in which the average person would rank various combinations of distress and disability. It was speculated that through a survey of people's opinions about a range of possible physical and mental states, knowledge could be gained of the 'normal' evaluation of quality of life (in ill health). At first it was not primarily intended to apply 'quality of life valuations' to guide resource allocation judgements in health care. For instance, an investigation in 1982 aimed merely to assess the credibility and consistency of British court awards for damages in personal injury.[99] This paper addressed the question:

> How does psychometric evidence from individuals on the **relative** values they attach
> to different states of (ill) health vary from person to person, and to what extent is
> the psychometric evidence consistent with the **relative** values implied in court awards?
> (p. 159).

To find an answer the authors made use of a (slightly adapted) map of 'ill health states' that two of them (Rosser and Kind) had developed during an earlier study. In this 'map' they combined four 'levels of distress' with eight 'disability states'. The 'levels of distress' were:

1. No distress.
2. Mild distress.
3. Moderate distress.
4. Severe distress.

And the 'disability states' were:

1. No disability.
2. Slight social disability.
3. Severe social disability and/or slight impairment of performance at work. Able to do all housework except very heavy tasks.
4. Choice of work or performance at work very severely limited. Housewives and old people able to do light housework only but able to go out shopping.
5. Unable to undertake any paid employment. Unable to continue any education. Old people confined to home except for escorted outings and short walks and unable to do shopping. Housewives able only to perform a few simple tasks.
6. Confined to chair or wheelchair, or able to move around in the home only with support of an assistant.

7. Confined to bed.
8. Unconscious.[99]

In the earlier study the investigators had asked 70 subjects – general and psychiatric nurses, medical and psychiatric patients, healthy volunteers and doctors – to rank six specific combinations of disability and distress. For instance they were asked: 'How many times more ill is a person described as being in state 2 compared with state 1?' A range of assumptions was explained, including the fact that the subjects' responses would carry two important implications:

    (a) The ratio will define the proportion of resources such as time of trained personnel, money, equipment etc. that you would consider it was justifiable to allocate for the relief of a person in the more severe state as compared with the less ill.
    (b) The ratio will define your point of indifference between curing one of the iller people or a number (specified by the ratio) of the less ill people.[101, quoted in 99]

Subjects were also asked to rank all other combinations of pain and disability, and then to place the 'state of death' somewhere on the scale of 'health states' they had just ranked. Rosser and Kind[101] converted their results to a scale on which 1.0 was said to represent 'normal health' (interpreted as no disability, and no distress) and 0.0 death (see Table 1).

Table 1. The Rosser and Kind health scale

			Distress	
Disability	A (none)	B (mild)	C (moderate)	D (severe)
1	1.00	0.995	0.990	0.967
2	0.990	0.986	0.973	0.932
3	0.980	0.972	0.956	0.912
4	0.964	0.956	0.942	0.870
5	0.946	0.935	0.900	0.700
6	0.875	0.845	0.680	0.000
7	0.677	0.564	0.000	−1.486
8	−1.028	—	—	—

Remarkably (not least because none of the respondents was in a position to make even the remotest empirical judgement about the nature of death) respondents ranked states 6D and 7C (confined to chair and in severe distress, and confined to bed but in moderate distress) as equivalent to death. Of the states better than death, they ranked only three lower than 0.845. All the others fell in the narrow range between 0.845 and 0.995.

A great many criticisms have been made of this technique. In particular its claim to portray typical values has been questioned on the ground that the sample was small, and hardly representative. Only six of the 70 participants were manual workers, 40 were professionals, and less than half had had experience of serious pain or illness. What is more, even given the woolly and strangely evaluative nature of the descriptions of the 'distress and disability states' ('housewives' and 'old people' were, for some reason, singled out for special attention), some of the survey's rankings are quite ridiculous. For instance, why should 'disability state 5' coupled with 'severe distress' (whatever this means) have been rated 0.700 while 'disability state 6' in 'severe distress' was rated 0.000 (likewise 6C, 0.680 and 6D, 0.000)?

Nevertheless, despite huge conceptual and methodological inadequacies, these results continue to form a substantial part both of the 'justification' and the suggested practice of the QALY assessment.[102] With the assignation of a value (1) to health, and with the conversion of states of ill health to ratios, health economists are theoretically enabled to 'modify' people's 'life years' to produce 'the quality adjusted life year' or QALY. Once manipulated in this way a life year 'adjusted for quality' and rated at, say, 0.900 can be said to be more desirable than a life year 'adjusted for quality' and rated 0.680. From this, it is a relatively simple move to consider what each QALY costs the health service. In this way, and when the cost is interpreted as money, five QALYs gained through a health service intervention at a cost of £10 000 constitute a 'better buy' than six QALYs gained at a cost of £18 000 since the 'cost per QALY' of the first intervention is £2000 and the 'cost per QALY' of the second is £3000 (assuming that the remaining £8000 could be used to generate more than one QALY elsewhere).

The Fundamental Problem with QALYs

It is clear that the QALY, like other health economic techniques, relies heavily on several assumptions. Furthermore, once the financial cost of therapies is incorporated into the computation, in order to facilitate judgements about the relative worth of medical therapies, then one further arbitrary element is introduced. Financial costs are not fixed, and indeed are often not set by the health service system at all. In capitalism costs can fluctuate (and can be manipulated) in a number of ways, and this is a most disturbing feature of any assessment of a therapy's 'cost per QALY'. If used in the hardest cases to choose who to treat and who not to treat, decisions will not be based solely on patients' assessments of their quality of life before and (potentially) after treatment, but will also take very substantial account of how much each therapy happens to cost.

But even this arbitrariness is not the essential problem. At rock bottom what is wrong with the QALY is that absolutely everything about it is arbitrary. QALYs do not really exist at all. They cannot be seen, they cannot be touched, there is not even the flimsiest guarantee that anyone conceives of QALYs in the same way as anybody else. What do you have in mind when you think of a QALY?

The QALY is a tactical, technical device necessary to allow one type of health economic system to function. But beyond the system there is no such thing as a 'quality adjusted life year'. Consequently, in reality, such measurements as 'cost per QALY' do not have meaning. Reference to this expression guarantees its existence no more than reference to 'cost per unicorn' guarantees a unicorn's existence. This is not to deny that different therapies produce different levels of active, enjoyable, or distress-free living. Of course they do, and if a therapy is shown to produce no benefit in a patient's ability to cope with life then this is the best possible reason to discontinue it. Conversely, those therapies which considerably enhance a person's life ought to be pursued, unless there are overwhelming reasons why not (and cost could be one). This much is fairly obvious, and has been obvious to genuine health workers throughout history. The QALY adds nothing to this basic health care purpose. It only appears to do so to insecure people who need to see numbers and measures to be convinced that something worthwhile is happening.

An Implicit Theory of Health

There is, however, one interesting feature of the QALY which is often overlooked. It is not strictly to do with the system itself, but with the implicit assumptions about the nature of health evident in its genesis. Study of the way in which the 'valuations of quality of life' were generated and analysed shows that, despite the apparently simple characterisation of health as 'no distress, and no disability', the general framework of the study is governed by a much broader theory. Of itself this is not particularly significant since the theory is not properly worked out (indeed no theory was intended), and there are many more rigorous and valuable analyses of health available. The real interest lies in the wider implications of the tacit endorsement of this theory in health economics, and ultimately in what this acceptance implies for the assessment of costs in health work.

Two related questions are of the greatest relevance:

1. What is the logical consequence of the health economist's interpretation of cost as sacrifice?
2. How did the studies which led to the invention of the QALY characterise the nature of health?

By themselves the answers to these questions are not compelling. They are merely indications that health economics is (idiosyncratically) heading towards a conclusion which is accepted by a growing number of philosophers (not to mention health care practitioners): that the effort to create health is not restricted to medical work (hardly anyone seems to think this nowadays), nor is it limited to the activities of the health service alone (currently very few express this opinion either).

The final (and much more interesting) component of this conclusion is that any realistic assessment of health care cost must take account of people's quality of life, and since this is so, health benefits and health costs cannot be confined to the health service sector alone. To regard these things as only of concern to the National Health Service is a quite artificial demarcation, both because considerations of quality of life extend beyond health service boundaries, and because the results of health service activity have direct implications for patients' future general life activities. Many people pay lip-service to this logic –

for example, those in the **Healthy Cities** movement who habitually recommend 'intersectoral collaboration for health' – but very few comprehend the ultimate implication for the health service as a whole.

The Four Stages of Cost-Assessment in the NHS

Once interpretation of cost is extended beyond the basic clinical notion (that is, that the human costs of sickness are limited to the suffering experienced as a result of medical conditions), then the **first stage** of NHS cost-assessment has already been passed. In the **second stage** there is detailed consideration of how money is spent within the health service, and how different NHS processes produce outcomes of different value at different sorts of cost. At the **third stage** there is talk about the wider social costs of the NHS – of the 'indirect costs' or the 'future costs' of the activities of health services on the 'gross national product' (GNP). But once this stage has been reached then it is inevitable that a **fourth stage** must occur. This stage has two essential features: (a) assessment of the benefits and costs (and effectiveness and efficiency) of medicine can no longer take place within the protection of the health service walls, and (b) the amount of state support made available to the traditional medical endeavour, as distinct from that given to other forms of social service (such as housing, education and public transport) must come under rational scrutiny. This, in effect, makes the problem over what is 'good' or a 'benefit' or a 'desirable outcome' a hundred times more fraught than it is now, where the debate is still by and large contained within NHS boundaries – but it is a necessary fourth stage if a more reasoned system of human care is to be established.

Health According to the QALY

Apparently unwittingly, by deciding to employ the ideas of 'distress' and 'disability' within their 'scale for valuing states of illness', Rosser and Kind built in an implicit theory of health. Although it has no philosophical grounding it nevertheless quite clearly extends the notion of health beyond clinical measurement and language. It is most important to recognise that their survey did not concentrate on clinical outcomes *per se*, or on the interpretation of outcomes viewed from a clinical perspective, but instead asked respondents to think about 'illness states' construed as **a range of possible levels of activity** (for instance, 'choice of work or performance at work very severely limited'). For the sake of the survey *illness* **was important only in so far as it was said to act to prevent people from doing things**, and medical interventions were important only in so far as they might be the means by which such 'illness states' might be relieved.

Thus, in the very way in which the foundation studies were set up, there is included a theory of health which is based on the express recognition of the ultimate importance of **people's ability to perform in life**. The problem of illness in Rosser and Kind's surveys (as in subsequent surveys[103]) was never the illness itself (which is merely an obstacle of a particular kind requiring a particular sort of intervention – sometimes a medical one) but rather what illness prevents people from achieving in their lives as a whole. Disease, illness, or 'ill health' is only one of very many possible impediments which can produce 'illness states'. Disease and illness are certainly possible causes of the problem but, as conceived by Rosser and Kind, are not the problem itself – or at least are only a contingent factor in the problem.

Cost as Loss of Autonomy

Essentially an illness is undesirable in proportion to the degree to which it inhibits people's autonomy, or movement in life (which is how Rosser and Kind's survey seems to understand it too). Therefore, the basic way to translate cost in health care is as loss of autonomy. Thus cost should not finally be understood as money, or even as the sacrifice of other possible clinical benefits – these are only initial comprehensions of the notion of cost. Ultimately, the cost of not having a problem treated (or solved) is not money (although it can mean loss of money), but **what a person is prevented from doing which he would find fulfilling**. It is quite clear from the choice of the framework and categories of their 'illness scale' that Rosser and Kind were thinking (probably unconsciously) of health in this sense (see two earlier works for a philosophical justification of the idea, and for a consideration of the limits of meaning and practice)[65,67]. If this is accepted then the common belief that **illness** is a central factor in the QALY method is obviously wrong. Illness just happens to be the debilitating factor Rosser and Kind assumed in their survey. What is important is not this conditional factor, but the framework (and implicit theory of health) itself. And this framework is based upon life outcome rather than clinical outcome, and so can be used for **any debilitating factor**.

To make this quite clear, if the 'distress and disability states' are not considered to be **necessarily** the outcomes of illness but 'outcomes in life' (and although Rosser and Kind described them as 'states of illness' such disabilities as 'being unable to undertake any paid employment' clearly may be produced in ways other than through illness) then **not only can problems beyond the concerns of medicine affect these outcomes but the QALY can be applied to consider the affect on quality of life of such life (or non-illness) problems as unemployment, boredom and educational deprivation**.

The Use of the QALY Beyond the NHS

If the above analysis is correct, and assuming – for the sake of argument only – that the QALY is meaningful, then there is no philosophical barrier to the use of the QALY to contemplate the relief of 'illness states' caused by impediments other than disease and illness. Consider, for a moment, the situation of

Christopher Smith, a 49-year-old senior lecturer at what used to be called Bramchester Polytechnic (now the Metropolitan University of East Central Bramshire).

Christopher is not a happy person. He finds his job boring and frustrating, he has to teach more and more students many of whom he is quite certain he is not helping in any way, and several of whom he firmly believes cannot benefit from the form of 'higher education' on offer at MUECB. Christopher once had hopes of following a lively academic career but soon found himself trapped by his expanding teaching and administrative commitments. Before long, and even though he was well aware of what was happening to him, he knew that he had sunk into a treacly mire of apathy. Now, nearly 20 years on, Christopher has no realistic chance of taking a job elsewhere, and very little hope of further promotion either. His head of department, who is several years his junior, is a quite recent appointment. He was undoubtedly given the post not as a result of any academic achievement (an increasingly irrelevant consideration in contemporary Higher Education – an enterprise which has quite deliberately been infected with NHSitis) but because he was seen as the sort of person who would gel well with the 'management ethos'.

Although it would not be correct to describe Christopher as 'ill' in any clinical sense he feels borne down with a sense of hopelessness, and a constant, nagging grieving for what might have been. He goes through the motions at work, while his sadness spills over into the rest of his life. Given this state of affairs it would undeniably be appropriate to place Christopher somewhere on the 'states of illness' map: he is distressed and he does have disabilities. Rosser and Kind's descriptions of the distress levels and disability states are too vague to guarantee any certainty about how Christopher's 'life years' should be 'adjusted for quality', but he might be considered to have anything from 'slight social disability' to 'choice of work or performance at work very severely limited', and anything from 'mild' to 'severe' distress (and so might be judged between 0.986 and 0.870 in Table 1).

In short, although not ill Christopher is, technically (according to the QALY framework), experiencing some sort of 'illness state'. He is less healthy than he might be and, if he is to be helped, the question is: what sort of intervention will afford the maximum relief of his 'illness state'? (A yet further question is: at what cost will such an intervention be justified?)

A Trojan Horse?

What Christopher's case means more broadly is that anyone who has some **distress** or who has some **disability** (even if it is only slight) can be said to be suffering an 'illness state'. What is more, since the **cause** of the illness states are not essential to the QALY assessment there is no reason why the use of the QALY should be confined to official health services. And this is a very important conclusion which, taken along with arguments advanced in other papers, has enormous implications for resource allocation, not only within the NHS but between the NHS and other systems which aim to enable people to live better lives. At a stroke a major conceptual protection of the health service crumbles away, and ironically the means of its destruction is implicit within a measure that many within the service would like to adopt if they could make it work.

I am not seriously suggesting that the QALY measure should be used to assess the costs and benefits of all potentially life-enhancing (or 'state of illness relieving') interventions. For example, I am not suggesting that the 'cost per QALY' of the State ensuring meaningful employment for all its members should be calculated and then set against the 'cost per QALY' of health service interventions to see which should be the priority. After all the QALY does not really exist, and is deeply flawed even as a technical abstraction. However, such a move is, within the framework of health economics, a quite proper extension of the use of the QALY.

To confine the QALY to the assessment of the merits of medical interventions alone is simply an arbitrary categorisation. That no-one seems to notice this is an indication of the powerful hold the health service still exerts over the minds of the vast majority of the British people, including the 'intelligentsia'. But, like the QALY, the NHS is a human creation which relies upon the acceptance of many logically unsustainable assumptions for its continued existence. If these assumptions are challenged then the notion of a separate service, with a special nature and special privileges (see Paper Four) begins to collapse. If this disintegration can actually take place (and certainly no compelling philosophical arguments exist which might be used in its defence) then really thoughtful open debate about the best way of using the nation's resources overall might take place as well. In such circumstances the NHS will not be seen as the only means by which to enhance 'quality of life' or to generate QALYs (which is, in any case, a very strange idea). Instead, advocates of more spending on health services will have to demonstrate that health service activity is cost-effective in the most fundamental sense of cost-effectiveness. In other words, following the conceptual demolition of the NHS defences it becomes vastly easier to begin reasoning free from the restrictions of taken for granted (but highly disputable) priorities. In these circumstances discussions on health policy might begin not with the demand for more for the NHS, but with a broad and novel question. Namely, out of all the ways at the disposal of this society to alleviate disability and distress, which are the most effective? Or to put the same question in another way: **which sorts of human effort will produce the greatest autonomy at least cost in loss of autonomy to others?**

The Logical Consequence of the Interpretation of Cost as Sacrifice

Although the idea that the truest notion of health care cost is 'loss of people's autonomy which might otherwise have been had' may appear inordinately general, it is not as far-fetched as it seems. In fact not only is the idea part of the make-up of the QALY, it is also the direct extension of another part of mainstream health economics.

Once the move is made to regard the NHS not as a closed system but as a part of a much wider and more complicated social network then the conclusion that 'health care cost = loss of human autonomy' is, sooner or later, inevitable. Most simply, just as the purpose of health work is not to tackle disease and injury as **problems in themselves**, but to confront them because of the human activity they prevent, so the effects of health services only **begin** with medicine. The ultimate point of health work is to place people in positions where they can continue to have meaningful lives, and so the ultimate effect of health work is, inevitably, very great.

Health economists are well aware that the effects of health work have implications beyond health service systems, but are naturally reluctant to include these costs and benefits within their deliberations, since even within the purely clinical sphere the task is well beyond the scope of their technical apparatus:

> . . . (should) the reduction of so-called 'indirect costs' . . . be counted amongst the benefits of a treatment in a cost-effectiveness analysis (ignoring here any technical difficulties that might arise in trying to do so)? The typical situation is as follows: earlier return to work, or less time spent off work . . . may increase national output and thereby benefit the community generally . . .

> It is sometimes claimed that a particular treatment 'pays for itself' because the increase in national output (decrease in indirect costs) that it brings about is larger than the service costs entailed (output used) in providing the treatment . . . A treatment which benefits the unemployable or the retired segments of the population generates no such additional benefits, nor will any such benefits show up for those whose (unremunerated) work is within the home. Even within the working population, this benefit will be greater for the highly paid than for the lowly paid . . . if the result of ignoring such changes [for reasons of ethics] is to concentrate treatments upon the non-working population, the resources available to provide health care and many other good things in life will be less than they might have been . . ..[104]

For many health economists, and certainly for Williams (note the reference to 'so-called' indirect costs, and the other uses of inverted commas), many of the conceptual barriers of the NHS already do not really exist. However, the implications of this insight are so daunting that for many it is difficult even to begin to contemplate them.

Part Three: Fortress NHS

Paper Six

Fortress NHS

As it is normally conceived the NHS is a bastion of principle and compassion besieged by a harsh world progressively starving it of essential supplies, but the real Fortress NHS is quite unlike its popular facade. In truth the several bulwarks which have been erected to protect the Fortress are only incidentally arrayed against the effects of hard times. As with any fortress the real point of its defences is to ensure that it, and its inhabitants, first continue to exist and second continue to be able to behave in the traditional way.[16,60,105] Of course the NHS is not entirely dominated by protectionism and self-interest, and a great many British people know, through personal experience, what good it can do. Few doubt that such services as accident and emergency, and palliative care, available to all people are an essential part of any civilised state (although it is also true that thoughtful criticisms of the efficacy of most other clinical disciplines can be found[106]). Rather, the objection is that the organisation has shut its doors firmly, and apparently permanently, against rational inspection, and this is not good enough in a society where most good things – not just medical services – are increasingly in short supply.

The Outer Walls

Fortress NHS is too enormous to capture fully in words, but the essential parts of its fortifications can be described. The outer walls of Fortress NHS are, as one would expect, the most obvious part of its shield. They are so conspicuous that it is hardly necessary to point them out, but for the sake of clarity they are made up of the following elements, most of which have been discussed previously. The key components of the outer structure of the Fortress are **mythology** (the continuing faith of the British people – most of them outside but some within – that the NHS is fully and coherently principled); the results of **political compromise** (both at the outset and throughout the development of the health service[107]); **hierarchy, internal regulations and discipline** (used – increasingly these days with the advent of the manager – to minimise both protest and innovation); and **professional and personal self-interest**[108] (disciplines and individuals benefit from working for the NHS and so have developed a range of methods to ensure that they continue to do so – a natural effect of which is the further protection of the system itself). In addition, outside the walls, but with generous access to the inner sanctum, there are perimeter strongholds. These lesser fortresses are peopled by those external to the NHS who have a strong financial interest in its continued and unimpeded existence. Pharmaceutical companies,[109] the manufacturers of other sorts of medical supply, and (increasingly) insurance companies and some legal establishments are the most common occupants of these strongholds. The drug industry in particular is a powerful ally, indeed some would say it is part of the fortress:

Prominent amongst medicine's ineffective methods is the use of drugs. The modern pharmaceutical industry explains its importance in terms of the demand it meets, the jobs it creates, the profits it makes and recirculates, the exports it sells, and last of all, the necessities it produces. The stream of 'new' drugs born as their predecessors' patents expire, of multiple variations on basic formulae, and of dazzling choices between virtually identical brands, makes the pharmaceutical industry more economically than socially useful. Yet the drugs industry completes the market relationship between doctor and patient, playing the role of wholesaler to the tradesman and his customer, and seeking to influence both in their decisions.

The prime target for the pharmaceutical industry is the doctor, and other health professionals (pharmacists, district nurses, health visitors) who can influence doctors. The doctor–drug company relationship is a cosy one, and much less uncomfortable than the doctor–patient relationship. One estimate put the cost of drug promotion for each GP as equal to the cost of paying a pharmacologist to retrain the doctor in the use of drugs for one month each year. A study in 1974–75 showed that GPs were then exposed to 1300 adverts for 250 different preparations, each month. In 1977 the drug companies spent £71 million on sales promotion, the bulk of it aimed at GPs. At 1979 prices, the average doctor can expect to have £30 000 spent on his or her 'postgraduate education' by the drugs industry – about twice the cost of his or her original education. Britain's 150 medical journals derive 40–60% of their income from drug company advertising, and 40 or so 'free papers', with frequency varying from weekly to monthly, are entirely financed by drug advertising. The pharmaceutical industry funds scientific and educational meetings, providing free food and drink and contributing to advertising costs and speakers' expenses, in return for promotional displays and the showing of advertising films.

The relationship works. In 1979 doctors wrote 370 million prescriptions for medicines costing £750 million, and the profits on the sales totalled £125 million. In 1980 the profit rate on drug sales to the NHS was 21%, with some companies showing nearer 30%. By comparison the pre-tax return for the chemical industry as a whole was 18.2%, and for all manufacturing industry it was 17.6%. Only advertising and oil were more profitable than drug production, and that was during a bad phase for the industry. (From reference 110, by permission.)

The outer protections of the Fortress have not been the subject of this collection of papers, but any conceptual analysis of health services must understand that they are there, or else remain abstract and impractical.

Inside the Fortress

In order to lend support to the outer walls (which have come under growing attack from a range of critics over the past 25 years – but have nevertheless remained intact) more subtle, partly concealed security systems have been installed. The illustration and explanation of these systems has formed the bulk of the present account, so it is unnecessary to add much further specific detail. However, it can be enlightening (particularly for the potential opponent or invader) to see these systems in context.

Much of the inner protection of the Fortress depends on the deliberate distortion of theories and definitions. That is, rather than rely solely on might, Fortress NHS has found it necessary to employ tactics which some might choose to describe as brainwashing. Less dramatically, it is clear at least that the defenders of the NHS have in recent years recognised the benefit of piling up further defences behind the existing wall of mythology. This set of defences is divided into four main types.

The first internal defence is the use of **special meanings** – where words which have well-known meanings in everyday life are given new and different meanings within the Fortress. This contortion of meaning is supported by the second defence, **the esoteric use of language**: not only are many technical terms used which are only accessible to the initiated – even though most might with only a little difficulty be translated into more common language – but technical language has in many circumstances come to be the only legitimate way in which to talk about health care processes at all. Also, since the use of technical language is generally more highly valued in the health service, it can be used as a trump card to override other priorities (such as being kind to people) which can be properly supported only by less technical language.[111]

The third inner defence is the deliberate **creation of an artificial framework**. This defence works by fitting prevailing circumstances into an artificial, man-made structure in order to ensure that the special meanings and use of language seem normal and not contrived. In this way it becomes possible to argue passionately against inequalities in health whilst accepting the considerable inequalities in wealth which prevail in present-day Britain. The contrived frameworks can have a quite numbing effect on the intellect, and can even make it appear reasonable that people are allowed to be jobless and homeless, and be generally neglected by the State, until they become sick. At which point a very great deal of money can legitimately be spent, to return them to a 'healthy misery'. Likewise, the creation of artefactual frameworks make it seem quite normal to claim that a person cannot need what the health service cannot supply her. Thus, artificial frameworks are designed to limit thinking and to prevent even the speculation that the Fortress may not be necessary.

Finally, and most obviously, **rhetoric is used incessantly**. This defence may not appear very astute, indeed it may seem more like a bludgeon than a sleight of hand, but its subtlety lies in the fact that after a while it ceases to seem to be rhetoric any more. Slowly but surely everyone begins to talk in the same way, as they unwittingly become more and more intellectually disabled. The nature of these defences may be further revealed by a brief review of their association with the 'four NHS principles'. This review also acts as a summary of key points developed in detail in the previous four papers.

Fortress NHS

Perimeter Strongholds (the protection of external interests – those companies who profit financially from the Fortress)

MYTHOLOGY

SPECIAL MEANINGS

PROFESSIONAL AND PERSONAL SELF-INTEREST

ARTEFACT

INCESSANT RHETORIC

POLITICAL COMPROMISE

'NEED'	'QUALITY'
Limited by NHS convention and systems – need is established from within the Fortress	Brazenly defined to give a quite different meaning to its meaning in the outside world. In the NHS quality is cheap
'EQUALITY'	'COST'
Prized by some defenders of the Fortress as a 'special principle' – but it can be sustained only with the help of other Fortress defences – an artificial category	Usually invoked as a way to limit spending. Health economists enlisted as defenders but this system works only within the Fortress – once the Fortress crumbles then so does this system

ESOTERIC LANGUAGE

HIERARCHY AND INTERNAL DISCIPLINE

Fig. 6

Need

As Understood within Fortress NHS

Within the Fortress 'need' or 'health need' cannot be any sort of need. Need is allowed to have meaning only within certain parameters. Here **what need can mean** is delimited by:

1. *Existing Services.*[112]
   It is simply asserted, as if there were no question about it, that:

   > these are our health services – if you have any health needs they must be for these things, if you do not need any of our services then you cannot have any health needs.

   What is more, the presence of such a vast collection of services gives massive credence to the view that such services simply must be needed. It is as if the boast were 'this is what is truly important – it must be, look at all the machinery we have in place for it'. It is very difficult to object to the use of so many services, especially where the majority of them are obviously useful. To suggest their replacement by other things of only potential use is, in every case, to propose a practical and political gamble which no one seems at all prepared to take.

2. *Experts*
   Those people with positions of authority and influence within the Fortress define, and in so doing limit, what can be needed. There is not necessarily any conspiracy to do this. Simply by doing the jobs they do, by using the often technical tools they use and in having the priorities associated with these jobs and tools, the various experts inevitably and constantly shape what is said to be needed.

3. *Disease*
   Where disease is seen as a primary evil, it becomes necessary to challenge it whenever it is encountered. In these circumstances the need for a cure is thought to be obvious, and does not require additional justification. Even though this need might conflict with other needs within the Fortress it must take precedence (such simple thinking is challenged more often today, not least as the result of heightened interest in ethics, but nevertheless remains a notable defence).

Clearly, the meaning of need is contrived within the Fortress.

As Understood in the Outside World

In the world at large anything lacking, from which benefit might be had if it were not lacking, might be said to be a need. In the world at large at its simplest a **need** is a gap between an actual state and a goal state, and is best thought of as a means towards the achievement of the goal in question – as a means of filling the gap. There are limits on the meaning of need in the outside world, but the set of things which **might be said to be needed** is not preordained in the way that it is within the Fortress. To give the most general example, in the world at large health is not always associated with disease or clinical priorities, and so it is not always possible to meet health needs solely by the sorts of service which are offered by the NHS.

Quality

As Understood within Fortress NHS

Within the Fortress care is taken to ensure that the meaning of quality remains obscure, but at the same time everyone within the health service is encouraged to use the word as much as possible, and literally forced to accept that a clear and proper definition of quality exists – somewhere. Great care is also taken not to set any clear standards for the 'quality processes' of the NHS since to do so would be to tie the hands of management unnecessarily.

Where reluctant attempts to define quality are forced the word is most commonly said to mean 'fitness for purpose'. What this means, of course, is that so long as there are 'customers' who are using whatever services there are, and 'their requirements' are being met, then (according to this definition) a quality service can be said to be in existence. So, as with need understood within the Fortress, what counts as quality inside Fortress NHS is established by what the existing service happens to offer to the 'customer' – that is, the very nature of quality is established by the Fortress itself, and on the terms of its occupants.

It is interesting to note further that several commercially inspired definitions of quality make quality dependent on meeting the needs of customers. Of course this is not nearly so generous and democratic as it appears since, through advertising and monopoly, business can itself determine what customers think they need. The NHS does not have this commercial power – very few people actually want to be hospitalised – and so is forced to use the more limited, and limiting, definitions of need summarised above.

As Understood in the Outside World

In the world beyond the walls of Fortress NHS, as people use the term in everyday conversation, quality is more usually equated with excellence. It is most unusual, in the ordinary world, to find quality being used to refer to 'that which is acceptable'. Good quality is commonly thought either to be something, or an aspect of something, which is above a certain standard. In real life good quality is routinely regarded as meaning 'something special'.

More generally, it is worth noting that the NHS distortion of the terms need and quality is produced primarily through the often intentional development of unconventional meanings for these words. In the cases of equality and cost however, the NHS relies not so much on the misrepresentation of language but on creating artificial, deliberately restricted circumstances and then permitting the use of these words only within those frameworks. Cost and equality are not 'allowed' to have meaning beyond certain spurious limits since this would stretch their interpretation – and their implications if applied – beyond what is useful to the Fortress.

Equality

It is frequently heard within the NHS – sometimes with genuine intent, and sometimes not – that equal access to services should be preserved at all costs, and that equality is an inviolable health service principle. However, not only is it clear that in practice equal access is not guaranteed in many circumstances, but the theoretical use of equality within the Fortress tends to be very vague. More than any other of the principles the espousal of equality in the health service relies on the acceptance of an assumed framework. Only if patients are considered separate from their general life circumstances – that is only if they are considered within an artificial situation where sickness is caused by 'bad luck' and medical services are special – can they be considered as equal. (To regard them all as 'equally human' and therefore of equal value is an argument with merit, but it is nonetheless itself a classic example of the creation of artefact by deciding to ignore all other differences which might at least be considered to be of relevance.)

It is very important to the maintenance of the Fortress that 'equality' continues to be used vaguely, for if the notion is taken seriously (as it is in Paper Four) it inevitably leads to the questioning of wider social inequalities. And once this becomes widespread the Fortress, and its resources, become endangered.

Cost

In the health service cost is either considered very crudely to mean 'the monetary price of activities', or it is seen through the models of health economics. These models offer a very clear demonstration that Fortress NHS protects itself partly through forcing the public to assume circumstances which do not really pertain. It is only by **imagining** the health service to be a largely self-contained system that the idea can seriously be entertained that 'internal markets' will work in the way that they do when normal conditions of supply and demand, and buying and selling apply.[83] And it is only if it is thought that the health service is an entirely self-contained system that it is possible to propose in earnest that the QALY might be used as a way to judge the relative value of health service activities. As soon as the many walls of the Fortress are seen to have no theoretical foundations, and to be the results of convention and deliberate manufacture (and so also to be remarkably vulnerable to an intelligent onslaught), the exclusive use of the QALY within the walls appears quite arbitrary. It is only because we have become so used to the presence and apparent strength of Fortress NHS, that no one has yet thought to ask why it is never suggested that the QALY should be used across the ramparts of the Fortress, rather than only within it.

Blanket Defence

In general, within the Fortress the meanings from the world at large are officially not thought or said to be legitimate. If it comes to the crunch they are simply not permitted – they may be ridiculed, they may be described as 'abstract' or 'esoteric', they may be crushed by hierarchy, or (which is still most common unless the advocate of the meanings is thought to be a 'trouble-maker' of some kind) they may simply not be heard by anyone that matters. Within the walls of the Fortress, thinking – if this is the right expression – is dominated by precedent, tradition, existing practice, contrived and distorted theory, vested interest and naked power. This, not reason, holds sway over what is done and over how what is done is justified (if justification is ever attempted). Yet outside the walls reason is still possible (even though there are many other fortresses out here). Outside Fortress NHS meaning exists free from NHS codes, familiar to most people as the sort of thinking used in daily living.

And so there is hope for those who envisage a different sort of health service – one far more open to debate and genuinely designed for the good of the people. The more conceptually disorientated Fortress NHS becomes, the more some of its inhabitants seek to bolster up the walls. And unfortunately for them even inside the Fortress they cannot build up all their battlements in secret, and – apparently conversely – the more they build the more they can be seen to be vulnerable. For example, the production of mission-statements is nowadays virtually an industry in itself (if 'mission-statement' consultants do not already exist it is surely only a matter of time before they do). There have even been suggestions from some 'management consultants' that the NHS should change its name. At the time of writing this has not yet happened, but it would not be a surprise if it did. For some people this concentration on words is taken to be a sign of progress towards a more up-to-date NHS with an impressive 'corporate image'. For others the attention to language rather than more substantial problems smacks of intellectual atrophy and despair, and is a telling sign of an age where far too many believe that expensive advertising can substitute for substantial planning. If this is indeed the truer view then it might – perhaps perversely – also be seen as a form of progress. Attention to superficial matters at the price of deeper reflection cannot go on for ever. Surely sooner or later sufficient influential people will come to recognise it for what it is, and then – without its facades or maybe because of them – the Fortress may begin to crumble.

Health Gain

The current most fashionable rhetoric (in 1993 at least) is the notion of 'health gain'. And with this latest development it might just be that saturation point has at last been reached.

It has already been seen that several health economists are coming to accept what some philosophers have known for years – that without a clear and applicable guiding definition of health much of their calculation and advice must remain abstract. The fact that health gain is being discussed in the various health service journals is an indication that this truth is slowly dawning beyond academia too. However, it is apparent that no one has any idea what best to do about this lack of conceptual guidance, and consequently the standard of the debate is consistently miserable. It is hard to imagine that conversation in the NHS can become more vacuous than it is over health gain, and the Fortress remain undamaged for much longer.

This is what the *Health Service Journal* (a magazine not normally noted for insistence on philosophical precision) wrote about health gain in August 1992:

> 'Health gain' is the catchphrase on every manager's lips. But what does it mean and how can it be achieved? . . . everybody (is) using the term 'health gain' (but there is) no clear definition of what it mean(s), how it (is) measured or what activities (lead) up to it . . .[113]

The *Journal* goes on to report one professor's definition of health gain as 'demonstrable improvements in health achieved through managed change', a statement which cannot possibly improve anybody's understanding since 'improvements in health' is just a different way to say 'health gain', as anyone can see.

The *Health Service Journal*'s feature was sparked off by the inauguration of new 'standing conference task groups' in Norwich and Belfast. Study of the background materials, and documents generated by the meetings,[114] gives an insight into the depth of the intellectual malaise which currently pollutes the NHS.

The 'briefing paper' to the Norwich Standing Conference[115] demonstrates that some within the service – at least those who are not yet wholly indoctrinated – are aware of the crisis. The document begins by announcing that despite the widespread use of the term health gain:

> . . . paradoxically, the first key issue is to lend some consistent meaning to the term itself, which is currently used rather imprecisely . . . Health gain is one of the new buzz-words of the nineties. Like so many buzz-words, it has no universally accepted definition, although sadly perhaps it is often used as the health equivalent of motherhood and apple-pie.

Those who have not explored the increasingly bizarre world of Fortress NHS may well be astonished that this vast, publicly funded organisation can permit such juvenile use of words in the first place, let alone fund standing conferences to discuss what 'technical terms' – which incredibly are already in use – might actually mean. However, the briefing paper goes on to express concern that if health gain means something like 'improving health status' (a term which is as vague as 'health gain', although because it has been around for longer no one worries much about it anymore[116]) then:

> it covers – even in this narrow sense – the **results** of the whole range of NHS activity, covering promotion, prevention, diagnosis, treatment, rehabilitation and continuing care.[115]

A little later on, a definition of health gain is bravely (or perhaps foolishly) hazarded:

> Health gain is the sum of benefits arising from the application of NHS resources to improving the health of the population and delivering quality health care to individuals.[115]

But, as the increasingly desperate tone of the article seems to concede, this leaves absolutely everything to be decided (connoisseurs of Fortress-speak may like to note an interesting empirical correlation – observed in the course of the present study – between the number of undefined words invoked to define yet more undefined words in health service articles, and the level of wretchedness apparent from the author's script). This is the health economists' problem, and so is the basic problem of all health service resource allocation: health work produces such a range of different classes of result that they cannot all be compared on the same scale, or even using the same techniques. At the root of it all, as always, is confusion about the meaning of health, and the lack of any meaningful common denominator even to begin to use it to bring all the disparate information under control. To his credit the author of the briefing paper is aware of this:

> . . . (definitions of health gain are) . . . too narrow if (they suggest) that we can consider 'technical' improvements to health status in isolation from other factors. In practice we do not generally do so, because in thinking about interventions we are usually also concerned with cost-effectiveness and appropriateness. Perhaps more to the point those who potentially might benefit from our interventions – patients, consumers, the population – do not see things in this way.
>
> These latter – surely the definitive judges – consider a wider collection of factors which together make up their personal and collective experience of the interventions made on their behalf. Thus access – in terms of geography, waiting time, even language and culture – is a vital consideration for most people, as is the issue of personal choice, or a greater degree at least of control over the circumstances of the healthcare they receive.[115]

But look at what is happening here. The author correctly explains that health gain, and therefore health, is a wide and varied notion which has different meanings for different people, and which – as he says – may have a different meaning for the doctor than it does for the patient. And so it surely follows from this reasoning that what is required is competent philosophical analysis of the meaning of health, at least to try to indicate which categories can be measured, which cannot, which may meaningfully be compared and which it is unfair to correlate. But, although analyses already exist – as do people with the capability and willingness to develop such analyses further – they cannot, for the many reasons outlined in these papers, possibly be contemplated within the Fortress.

Fortress NHS is rigid, irrational overall, and protected in a wide range of ways. Those people seeking genuine developments within it (as the author of the paper in question seems to be) are trying, probably without intending it, to work out ways to change the system. But they cannot possibly succeed for their success would be to make the Fortress unstable. The very last thing the defenders of Fortress NHS want is to let in reason from the world outside, so the very last thing they can allow is the unfettered, disinterested analysis of health for this would mean that there would sooner or later have to be clarity about health service purpose. Thus, there is a classic stalemate – those outside cannot get in to effect change, and those inside have no wish to get out.

So, in the briefing document, and in countless similar costly documents which litter the desks of NHS staff, rather than do the only sensible thing, it is necessary to adopt an alternative strategy. In the case under study the way forward was seen to be to list some 'main development priorities' which it is said:

> are already beginning to be addressed in the NHS, and are needed in any case, not only to achieve health gain, but to secure best overall value for money, and to respond effectively to the needs and wishes of consumers.[115]

Among the list of 'key areas for development' are included:

- techniques for the **assessment of need**, which are systematic, comprehensive, make effective use of available information (including that in primary care), and reflect the expressed needs and wishes of users and carers . . .
- a continuing search for a **better balance of services**, with the aim of releasing resources (capital, revenue and human skills) for reinvestment in **new more appropriate patterns of care**
- **better use of resources** measured in terms of outputs as well as outcomes
- a management discipline of **targeting for results**, requiring effective planning, implementation and control of performance
- the effective **involvement of consumers** in assessing needs, determining priorities, defining desired outcomes . . .[115]

and so it goes on.

No lack of respect is intended for the efforts of the author, or for those of other people who are genuinely – although vainly – struggling with the conceptual disaster that the NHS represents; but without proper, prior philosophical spadework their task is simply hopeless. Many of the reasons for this judgement should by now be obvious – need is not a single notion but has plurality of meaning; a 'better balance of services' requires first a justified account of what a 'better balance' might be, and second a precise practical description of this balance and its daily operation; 'targeting for results' requires distinctions between good and bad, and better and worse results, and also requires some way of judging between different categories of result so as to enable a manager to say 'for these reasons, on this month, I target X as a priority rather than Y'; 'involvement of consumers', if it is to be at all meaningful, requires a massive practical commitment to both general and NHS specific education so that consumers will be able to 'assess needs, determine priorities, and define desired outcomes' (and the size of this task could not be better indicated than by the utter failure of the full-time professionals in this endeavour).

So long as Fortress NHS exists these goals cannot be achieved. Unless there is clarity of purpose there cannot be any theoretical clarity in policy-making. Without hard thinking about which principles should inform the work of the health service, which variant of each principle is the most sound, and how this detailed theory can actually shape practice no theoretical progress is possible. At the very least, the size of the task must be recognised.

Clearly things have got out of hand. If managers cannot even develop the most elementary conceptual tools the NHS is in a parlous state, where things still 'just happen',[117] where powerful people get what they want, and where the idea that the NHS is democratic in any meaningful sense of the word is simply laughable.

Dialogue Three

Frustration

It is Friday morning. Melanie and the philosopher are sitting by themselves at a table in the busy basement canteen of the hospital.

Melanie:. . . The trouble is I don't see how your papers can possibly help me in the meeting today – your ideas are not specific. You are in no better position than the author of the 'health gain' paper. You don't have 'clearly worked out coherent principles which can be applied to guide practice' either, do you?

Philosopher: No, it is fair to say that I am not yet in a position to offer that much to you. I'm not even sure that what you are asking for is theoretically possible. If the successes of health care are so rich and varied it is foolish to look for a simple way of assessing them all. However, I don't agree that I'm in the same position as you and your colleagues.

For one thing I believe that I understand the problem and the reasons why it is a problem much more clearly than you do, so if there are solutions then I'm much better placed to find them. Secondly, I am in a position to outline a range of options for resource allocation and health service reform from which you might choose, and I do have my own preferences which I can at least partly justify by pulling together some of the conclusions of my analyses of the principles. For instance, if you take quality seriously rather than rhetorically then the current trend for 'management-led' quality assessment – or whatever the jargon is – is simply untenable. And what's more, I do think I have found a common denominator which we might at least discuss. If it turns out to have some plausibility then you have a great deal to think about, and potentially the basis for many arguments to change health services for the better – not just this hospital.

Melanie: Okay, perhaps you are not exactly in the same boat as some of the other people who are thinking and writing about the health service, but you are still talking far too generally. You are being paid by the service you know, so you had better bear in mind that people will be expecting you to produce results.

Philosopher: I appreciate that, and I want to do what I can. You wanted me to tell you whether or not it is ethical to shut your geriatric ward?

Melanie: Yes, but after reading your papers I now feel that everything is now so complicated that proper decision-making (as you would call it) is completely beyond us and that we **would** be better off drawing straws. I know you are opposed to the politics and power games of the 'Fortress', but this is how we get answers (imperfect as they may be) – and the health service does still manage to do a great deal of good. Perhaps what we have is the best we can realistically hope for? I'll bet you that Dr Graham gets his way today whatever I or anyone else says.

Philosopher: But that's fatalistic. You are giving in to the pressure of the Fortress, and I know you think the geriatric ward should be spared. Surely you don't want to report back to the full committee with a recommendation that everyone should continue to fudge and fiddle?

Melanie: No, I don't. But I need you to give me some help.

Philosopher: I could be of most help if it were possible to work on a radical reassessment of the health service – to design a philosophical reform of health care.

Melanie: But you know enough to know that this is impossible.

Philosopher: No. I am optimistic enough to think it is a very slim possibility. I think much depends upon whether or not the philosophy of health develops into a mature discipline, and whether those in charge of the NHS develop real techniques to address their philosophical problems. I admit that at the moment there is a very long way to go with this. But it is not impossible. I have not argued ideas which are too complicated or esoteric for people to grasp. All I have done is to display the depth of the principles.

Melanie: It is very frustrating. I do see the logic of your arguments but they do not fit with what I know of the real world. I cannot possibly explain all this to the committee, and I certainly don't think that you should appear before them again.

Philosopher: I am frustrated too. I know that my analyses, and the further suggestions I have here (*he picks up his final paper*) have profound difficulties, but I'm afraid this is simply inevitable. I am at least offering a general justification for a health service rationale where none exists at presert. The alternatives to my analysis are theoretically much less elegant, indeed they are very confused and tend to leave people's fate to chance.

Melanie: Yes, but there are significant and very unpalatable consequences of your theory, as you have already described it, which fall into the realm of ethical controversy. If you shift national resources in the way that you are hinting with your preference for an 'equalising' policy – combined with your views that 'Fortress NHS' can act against the provision of broader social welfare – many people who are now treated expensively by medicine will no longer be entitled to that treatment, and you will also curtail many advances in medical research which might eventually prove to be of great benefit. You can't ignore these difficulties. What you suggest might mean that some very sick people will be turned away from health services.

Philosopher: What you say is true, assuming the same amount of government funding, and it is rightly part of the overall problem. It is not easy, and there is a big price to pay for my overall solution, although I do have some provisional answers to it which I outline in the final paper. Roughly though, my theory is based on the single basic idea of ensuring decent levels of autonomy first for everyone in society, and then, when those conditions have been provided, to work to raise the levels of autonomy of those who – for whatever reason – fall below this general level. What I mean by autonomy is not only the freedom to be able to make choices, although that is important, but the freedom to be able to do creative things in life. So, what I mean by welfare provision is not just unemployment and other financial social benefits, but continuing education, worthwhile work, and the constant opportunity for general personal development (and not just for the majority or the 'normal' members of a society but for everyone, including the very handicapped and the very sick). It is already true today, in many cases in Britain, that sick people could have been helped to live longer if uncontrolled spending on medical advances had been allowed in past years. What my proposal will mean, by redistributing some resources from within the Fortress to the wider world, is that more sick people will die earlier than they otherwise would. And this, I agree, is hard to stomach. But on the other hand a great many more people will have more fulfilling lives, will enjoy free and communal leisure facilities, will have jobs to do, and will be supported in a range of ways in which they are not now. Given the mass of evidence that better lives tend to mean longer lives too, the medical profit and loss may balance out. The difference with my proposal is that it is based on a coherent philosophy rather than left to variables such as market forces, age, and place of abode.

How will these ideas affect the decision to be taken in your Trust? Well, if I had the power to make the changes I would like to see, the decision would almost certainly not lie with you at all, but would be taken by the old people concerned, within the welfare options which had been generally agreed within society. What would be crucial would not be their length of life, nor necessarily even the continuation of every medical treatment, but the size of their capacity to live a life which fulfilled them. What this would mean would be that each person would have to be very carefully consulted, and, within the range of general social provision would be enabled to decide – with necessary assistance – what they might do. Some may prefer to live within a closed community (or institution), others with friends, others on their own with support from health services. And the goal of the health services would be, in the first place, to achieve as much fulfilment as possible before any other priority. Now this would of course mean that medicine in many cases would still take a key role, but that role would always be subsidiary to **overall purpose**. The health service would not, in other words, operate as it does now and direct itself in all the many different ways I have discussed so far. In other words the external drives, and the drives associated with maintaining the Fortress, would be dismantled and superseded by drives based on creating and sustaining the foundations necessary for a fulfilled existence.

It would not have to mean the end of medical research though it might mean that there would be less money available for such research, and that researchers would have to demonstrate how their work might be of use in the increase of people's capacity to do fulfilling things in life. It would also mean that there would be more research into better ways of welfare provision, and more projects to devise and assess new ways of enabling people in a more general way. For example, rather than invest money into massive epidemiological studies of some screening programmes money might be invested into trial schemes to provide free, clean, safe and efficient public transport in various areas of the country, or spent on the study of human happiness – and how best to achieve it. The pay-off of such schemes could be tested in terms of morbidity and mortality – in the time honoured medical manner – and also for a wider range of costs and benefits (the QALY could be used here – if anyone wanted to use it – just as it is occasionally used within traditional health care assessment).

Melanie: But people would die in pain if you withdrew some of the more expensive or specialised medicine. There would be one hell of a fuss.

Philosopher: People often die with one pain or another anyway, but more pain is not necessarily a consequence of what I suggest. People in pain tend to be very disabled and not autonomous so pain control would be a priority. It is also true that by prolonging life through successive medical interventions when the chances of recovery are slim more pain is produced over a longer period of time. You are right that there would be one hell of a fuss, but this fuss would have to be laid out on a broader canvas along with other fusses over people starving on this planet, or over people committing suicide because life is so hopeless, and people living pointless lives because the facilities do not exist for them to do something more creative.

I'm sticking my neck out to say it's time that we thought about what we want and time to take the courage to stop doing some things which we are currently doing simply because we have got used to doing them. Britain is a deeply conservative society where traditions are very hard to break. It is not necessary to be opposed to the intellectual and practical stagnation and decline such traditions bring to see that, in such a society, we must take the utmost care before we establish future precedents. Currently genuine health reform is prevented by the 'it's possible' argument. This may sound very positive, but what it amounts to is the Fortress claim: Look, we can do this, it's possible. We cannot therefore even suggest that we might actually stop it in order to replace it with a better possibility.

Melanie: Perhaps you are right, but people would die earlier, there would be pressure on people to commit euthanasia, there may even be the sorts of pressures some Americans are discussing to force people to 'die cheaply'.

Philosopher: These sorts of pressure come about only in the world where the Fortress exists – they occur only because medicine is seen as a special case when in fact this position cannot be sustained theoretically. Break the Fortress down, establish clear social welfare priorities based upon a philosophy to create autonomy, then these issues dissolve and are replaced by open planning.

Melanie: I think you are a hopeless idealist.

Philosopher: I have ideals, certainly. However, I am trying to think the problem through rationally and steadily, to see if this method can produce more consistent thinking and decision-making about people's health. Please read my last paper. I know better than anyone that it does not contain truly substantial answers, and that there is much more work to be done yet. But I can outline some options for you, and I can at least begin to describe the sort of philosophical framework under which serious planning for health should take place.

Paper Seven

Options

Introduction

In theory the NHS might be changed in an almost indefinite number of ways, and for a variety of reasons.

Two key grounds for change have emerged out of this series of papers: the need to ration and the need to reform the system as a whole. Clearly these reasons may be related, and one motivation might naturally have an effect on the other, but they are not necessarily associated. New measures to ration health care may have no impact on the basic nature of the health service (certainly the rationing schemes implemented to date have had no such fundamental effect[25,26]), and reforms to the system need not be inspired by any perceived need to ration. Furthermore, rationing and/or reform to health services might take place either within the present confused health service rationale, or outside it – under an alternative *raison d'être* – although any changes made in the former case will be relatively minor.

Seen in this light, the following possibilities exist:

1. Ways to arrive at fairer methods of resource allocation (or rationing) within Fortress NHS might be suggested.
2. Ways to reform the internal structure of Fortress NHS might be proposed. Such proposals may or may not change the distribution of specific medical services.
3. Proposals might be advanced for the allocation of medical services if Fortress NHS were dismantled.
4. A broader framework for health work, one which assumes that the walls of Fortress NHS have been broken down, might be outlined.

Option 2 falls within the realm of 'health service administration' and is precisely what every previous 'reform' of the NHS has tried to do, always with the aim of controlling financial cost. As such it is the tinkering option. It does not address the heart of the problem because it does not address the question of purpose, and there is no point in discussing it further since its many practical weaknesses have made themselves apparent over the years, and its conceptual flaws have been exposed throughout this collection of papers.

Options 3 and 4 may be combined in order to keep the analysis within reasonable limits. Contrary to the views of those who regard medical services as simply part of the market, like any other service which might be bought and sold, most medical activity is best thought of as a sub-set of health services[65] and, following any dismantling of the Fortress, would need to be organised as part of broader health service provision. Medicine is not a 'discipline apart' (despite what so many doctors have been told in medical school), and it is quite artificial to debate the role and allocation of the work of medically trained people without taking into account wider social considerations. If it is believed that health services do have a special character, and that medical services are a proper part – but only a part – of health services (as I believe), then how much of what sort of service should be provided becomes a matter for deep and sustained public deliberation – a matter of planning rather than gambling on the market.

Thus, only two general approaches to change are considered in this final paper. These are:

1. The suggestion of ways to arrive at fairer methods of resource allocation (or rationing) within Fortress NHS.
2. The suggestion of a broader framework for health care, assuming that the walls of Fortress NHS can be and have been broken down.

PART ONE

Rationing Within the Fortress

While considering options for rationing under the conventional understanding of health services it must always be remembered that many of the alternatives which might be thought fair within the Fortress will carry with them the special understandings and assumptions of the Fortress. Many types of 'fortress fairness' may be only artificially fair since people's life circumstances tend to be considered only in a limited fashion within the health service.

In Britain, over the past 10–15 years, health economists have taken the lead in the debate about how best to ration scarce health service resources. For the most part they have been concerned to develop proposals for the 'rational allocation of resources' within the Fortress but, as has already been seen, if the logic of their ideas is pursued fully their suggestions inevitably spill over the walls. A survey of contemporary work reveals that quite a number of options for rationing have been seriously considered, very few of which seem to have been absolutely ruled out. Most are interesting, some controversial, but as yet none has been substantially analysed.

Contemporary Options for Rationing

The Use of Ethical Principles

The consensus amongst British economists at least is that however many – or few – 'basic ethical principles' are produced they will not be sufficiently clear to guide tough health service decision-making. As an example Alan Williams gives the choice of the Stanford University Medical Centre Committee on Ethics, which is: preserve life, alleviate suffering, do no harm, tell the truth, respect the patient's autonomy, and deal justly with patients. Health service literature has been inundated with such phrases in recent years, and Williams is undoubtedly right to dismiss most of them as impractical, at least in the way they are normally presented. It is extremely unlikely that the highly complex processes of caring for people where resources are scarce can be brought under control simply by such advice as 'do no harm' and 'alleviate suffering'. However, just because this sort of thinking cannot solve the problems it takes on, it is not therefore rendered entirely useless. It is possible to use these principles as a way in to deeper deliberation, and they can certainly form part of structures within which individual health workers can think. However 'ethical principles' such as these are clearly too ambiguous and open to interpretation to be used for the purpose of rationing health services consistently.

Williams is equally scathing about appeals to 'egalitarianism' as a principle of rationing. He thinks that when hard rationing choices have to be made it is hardly sufficient for 'ideologists' simply to assume as a matter of record that the NHS should be 'egalitarian'. For Williams there can be no 'moral ought' about egalitarianism if its proponents cannot express their beliefs in a way which might be usefully applied to the organisation of health care. For this economist:

> An egalitarian stance pervades . . . alternative systems, though . . . (it) . . . is not sufficiently well specified to offer clear guidance to analysts as to what the distributional policy of the system actually is.[91]

However, Williams has set up an easy target. In Part Two of this paper it will be seen that an egalitarian notion can be meaningfully applied to the 'distributional policy' of health work , at least to suggest a general, purposive framework within which more specific decisions might be made. Egalitarianism is so 'unspecified' at present firstly because the philosophy cannot be consistently applied within the NHS for practical reasons and secondly because thinking is restricted by the artificial constraints described previously.

Setting Specific Limits on Medical Therapy

Although it has not yet been seriously proposed as an option for the NHS, in the US – where different mythologies hold sway – a number of credible commentators have gone to print to propose that the State should set clear limits on what medical problems should and should not be treated, and on the range of treatments which might be used. In some articles it is merely the medical conditions and therapies which come under scrutiny, in others it is the worth of the patients themselves.

It must be noted that the American health system is very different from the British health service. Most Americans pay for their medical services through private insurance, and only the elderly and those in poverty are normally eligible to receive medical help through state provision.[30] Government help for medical services is severely limited, which partly explains the high level of attention which rationing policy has received in the US.

Oregon, a state in the north west of America, has received much publicity for proposing (and, to date, partly undertaking) an experiment in which the medical services available to those people eligible for Medicaid[118] are rationed according to a 'formula' which takes account of public perceptions of the relative importance of treatments, clinical judgements, 'quality of life' and the money available to the state for spending on medical services. Part of the formula allows the state to establish a 'league table' of therapies (there are currently 688 in all).[87] Depending on the way the formula works out in any financial year the number of treatments which the state will fund is set. All people eligible for Medicaid may receive any of the treatments above a 'funding line', if this is judged to be clinically appropriate, but below the line the treatments simply are not on offer.

Although many find such a scheme offensive (for instance, it is often objected that if you are rich or well insured in Oregon you can have whatever treatments are on sale) it does not discriminate between identified individuals, and does not – at least in principle – take into account the 'worth', or the way of life of the people who might benefit from medical treatment. However, there are plenty of schemes around which do advocate precisely this sort of discrimination.

Perhaps the two most well-known proposals of this sort are those of Daniel Callahan[119] and Paul Menzel.[120] Both writers suggest that because US spending on medical services takes up so much more of the nation's domestic product than it does in other countries radical measures are required to keep it in check. Both too are concerned that spending ever more money to keep sick people alive for ever longer cannot help but have a detrimental impact on the lives of other Americans. Callahan focuses in particular on the 'greying population'. The life expectancy of America's elderly continues to increase, and this tends also to mean greater dependency on the state.[121] Callahan argues that unless the costs of geriatric care are kept in check younger and more productive Americans will suffer.

The answer to this, according to Callahan, is to set an age limit on eligibility for Medicare. Beyond a certain chronological period no treatment should be offered to those who cannot pay for it. His thinking is not as harsh as it sounds on first hearing, and he gives a number of plausible arguments in support of his case (for instance, old people may not necessarily want to go on living, many will have had a full life, and some treatments do not produce more fulfilling life – just more life). In earlier writings Callahan was reluctant to say what this age limit should be, and he also allowed for exceptions to his rule to provide for circumstances where an old person seems especially productive or energetic, but now he is clear that there should be one set age limit for all.[122]

It is easy to be critical of this suggestion but, if one thinks of **cost as sacrifice** it becomes clear that not to suggest any reasoned way of managing an out-of-control situation is hardly morally better than Callahan's idea, and by abrogating responsibility is arguably worse. However, it should also be borne in mind that Callahan's argument accepts a blatantly **artificial** situation where there is one sort of care available to the rich and another sort available to poorer people (up to a point). If it is accepted that one of the reasons for poorer people's sickness might be the other hardships they have had to bear in life, then his discussion can seem much less reasonable.

Menzel goes further than Callahan. For many of the same reasons as his colleague Menzel accepts the need to find clear ways to ration medicine, but he extends the notion of 'worth' further. For Menzel it is plain that some people are not worth treating because they are a drain on society. Even if they get better they will offer nothing back to the community, therefore it is in the general public interest that they are denied help if they cannot afford it. Menzel even goes so far as to say that at least some classes of indigent people have 'a duty to die cheaply', and in so doing echoes the bar-room sentiments of America's still colonialist right-wing. Even more outrageously, he claims that study of the spending habits of poverty-stricken people show that this is what they prefer. The 'logic' is that people's spending patterns are a more reliable indicator of their stated preferences and values. Surveys show that 'the poor' prefer to spend their money on food and entertainment rather than invest in medical insurance. Therefore they put less value on their lives than those people who invest in 'health insurance plans'. In Menzel's own words:

> If one is poor one will certainly prefer to spend less on preserving health and saving life than if one is well off, even if in either case one is perfectly knowledgeable and rational. People of different means will quite properly choose differently when it comes to making use of statistically very expensive or marginally beneficial procedures. To flatten out these differences through uniform health-care services without changing the basic distribution of income would seem to ride roughshod over people's preferences for the different respective lives they have to live. Even if the difference in their preferences is largely a function of unjust inequalities in wealth among them, why should the rational choices of poorer persons be overridden?[120]

It is not important to defeat this argument here, indeed it is to be hoped that ways of questioning it are obvious. However, whilst it is not necessary to enter into a debate with those Americans who take the view that medical services are commodities like any other, it is important to discuss similar – although as yet a little more moderate – views which are gaining popularity in Britain.

Rationing Health Service Resources on the Grounds of 'Personal Merit' and 'Responsible Behaviour'

It has already been seen that health economists are aware of the importance of taking the 'indirect costs of health care' into account. The logic is that to ignore these effects (perhaps out of a combination of 'clinical duty' and the notion that health care is special), and to concentrate treatments on the least productive people, is effectively to reduce the resources which might be generally available both for health care and other good things in life.

This way of looking at things fosters the view that individuals are responsible to the community in two ways: they should contribute to it if they can, and they should not behave in ways which make it likely that they will damage its wealth. It follows from this view that behaviours such as smoking, and drinking too much alcohol, may 'carry the penalty' that if there has to be rationing the claims of the 'irresponsible person' will be heard only after those of the responsible (healthy living) person. Such arguments are now quite often advanced in writings in health promotion and education,[123] and have been supported by small-scale surveys[94] which suggest that people agree that non-smokers should be treated in preference to smokers, and light drinkers before heavy drinkers.

Rationing through 'Economic Productivity'

It has also been suggested by some British academics that, again because health service costs cannot logically or practically be confined solely to the NHS system, if it is necessary to ration health care then preference should be given to those people who are most economically productive. This way, once treated, the energetic not only produce benefits for themselves but, through taxation, also contribute to the more general good of the nation. On this way of thinking it becomes conceivable[91] that a QALY should no longer be a 'neutral measure', where a 'life year adjusted for quality' is of equal value no matter who has it, but should be further adjusted to take account of a person's general 'lifestyle'.

Market Options

It has been increasingly suggested in recent times that the way to keep health service costs under control is to introduce competition to foster efficiency.[124] The introduction of 'the market' into health care has been the subject of often heated debate elsewhere,[125] and whether or not markets can do what their advocates claim is beyond the scope of this analysis. However, it may be helpful to note that strategies 2, 3 and 4, which were listed in Paper Four (see p. 78), might be considered if it is thought appropriate to think of patients as the 'buyers' of care.

The Use of Lottery

This option is sometimes suggested in desperation, after hope of establishing a coherent alternative has been abandoned. The idea is that where there can be no fairness the best arbiter is chance. However, this option seems irresponsible in the very worst sense. In effect, to take this option is to refuse to accept responsibility for difficult decisions, to embrace even patently absurd results, and to eschew serious deliberation. What is more, any proposed lottery must take place within the confines of the NHS:

> . . . lotteries do not spring fully formed from Heaven. They are invented by people. These people have to decide who is eligible to enter this lottery, what the prizes are, how soon and how often you can re-enter this lottery if you fail to win the first time, whether tickets (especially winning tickets) can be traded or given away, and so on . . ..[91]

Lotteries would, therefore, be a clear case of the creation of artefact within the Fortress.

Democracy

To involve the people of a nation in decisions about the nature of a public service (if this is what the NHS is) seems to be a moral requirement. On the face of it the onus should fall on those who would not involve the public to give reasons why not, rather than on democrats to give an account of why they should. But the fact is that at present very few people outside the health service (and a great number within it too) have no say at all about what happens to it.

Many of the reasons for this are clearly to do with the wish of powerful people to maintain their power. But beyond selfishness it is true to say that a great deal of effort would inevitably be required to erect systems to involve people meaningfully in the determination of NHS policy. In order to involve the public in rationing decisions in any serious, practical manner it would be necessary, even purely at the level of theory, to establish:

1. The degree of participation thought sufficient.
2. The degree of knowledge required of:
   - the treatments
   - the context of the health service in which treatments are to be provided
   - the conditions which are to be treated.[87] People will have to be asked to judge the importance of situations and conditions which they have not experienced. And one has only to think about a time in which one found a new experience surprisingly pleasurable – or surprisingly difficult – to understand what a considerable problem this is.
3. The extent to which people must be impartial.
4. How the questions should be asked – to ask for a choice between treatment A and B is different from asking people to choose between person A and B, and different again from asking about a choice of services across the range of welfare provision rather than within the Fortress only.
5. Whether people should be asked to vote for systems, or ways of decision-making in general – or whether there must be some way of arranging continued consultation about a range of specific issues.
6. Whether majority agreement could be considered a form of 'social contract'.

The Oregon experiment in the US[87] and other lesser surveys have already amply demonstrated the extent of the difficulties involved if democracy is sought.

PART TWO

A Principled Framework

The suggestion of alternatives to an unsatisfactory situation is by far the hardest part of any complex analysis. The present case is complicated by three additional difficulties, the first of which is that if no answer is submitted to the management problem which prompted the inquiry, then the accusation of 'dodging the issue' is inevitable. The second difficulty is that if a solution to the managerial problem is proposed then by its very suggestion the solution will take for granted everything which the analysis has tried to deny. If it is true that the application of reason can have only a limited effect within Fortress NHS, and if it is also true that to think within the Fortress at all implies the acceptance of arbitrary and artificial categories, then any such proposal will confirm the madness which brought about the problem in the first place. The third complication is that if instead of offering a specific answer to the dilemma it is proposed to change the very circumstances in which it came about, without doubt the charge will be that the recommendation is unreal and idealistic. Thus all possible paths seem to be undermined. But this is the price which one expects to pay for choosing to take such a perplexing problem seriously.

With the above pitfalls in mind this paper does not offer a straightforward answer to the question: *should the geriatric ward be closed down?* This is not to say that I do not have preferences, or that there are no answers. Clearly there are many – any of the options described in Part One might be adapted to provide a solution, if so wished (in Callahan's view,[119] for example, the managers might conclude that the old people are simply no longer entitled to medical help).

Abolish the NHS

Instead, this final part of the investigation offers the suggestion that the wholesale, philosophical reform of the NHS is necessary, and in so doing concludes that the service must be dismantled – that it is time to abolish the NHS. It is argued that by taking each of the four 'basic principles' seriously, and by combining their most convincing and compatible aspects, a far better basis for a planned welfare and medical service is available (whether it is politically possible is another matter). Unlike what exists, the suggested system does have a basic common denominator of success, and could be used – within an alternative practical set up – as a general guide to health care decision-making. No set of general principles can ever be sufficient for, or take the place of human reasoning and judgement.[126] Such processes will always be necessary for the consideration of specific problems. However, a guiding system can work to define the range of legitimate solutions. Dependent on the particular framework in place, what may or may not be done within it may be quite different. As things stand, the management group is extremely restricted in its options by the towering presence of Fortress NHS.

The Purpose of Health Care

The shape of any framework to guide health services ought to be determined by a theory of health care purpose. The view outlined below offers an indication of one such theory, but does not enter into fulsome philosophical detail. Such detail is, however, available elsewhere.[65,67,127]

In principle the purpose of health care is absolutely simple. In every genuine case of health work the purpose of the worker must be to increase the autonomy of the person or persons who are being cared for. If, in the process, the autonomy of the health worker is also increased, so much the better. The means towards the creation of additional autonomy is always the removal or reduction of one or more obstacles which stand in the way of people achieving fulfilling potentials in life.

In order to understand the conceptual basis of the proposed post-Fortress framework for health services it is vital not to be confused about the essential nature of autonomy. At bottom a person with some degree of autonomy is able to control at least part of his world, the person without autonomy is powerless, and no-one is omni-autonomous. Obstacles such as disease, ignorance and injury can impede a person's autonomy. The basic task of health workers is to minimise these, and other obstacles, wherever they occur and wherever the worker has the necessary skills, unless to do so will disempower the person in question more. The success of health work, on every imaginable occasion, is indicated by the extent to which a person's level of autonomy has been increased. Whether the 'health outcome' is a growth in understanding, freedom from infection, the relief of pain, or the cure of injury it can only be judged a success if the person on the receiving end can do more in life as a result. If she cannot, if on balance she is disabled by the intervention, then it will simply not have been a health intervention.

Of course, this **common denominator** does not, for instance, offer specific help in deciding whether or not to invest in a screening programme rather than in more staff at a health centre, where these investments offer very different types of increased control. Nor is the denominator on its own of help in deciding whether it is better to increase the autonomy of one person rather than another. However, it does at least provide common ground for the comparison of alternatives and, once the notion is coupled with other principles of health care, can offer a substantial means by which to arbitrate in many difficult dilemmas.

Most significant of all, if it is accepted that health work has the basic goal of enabling people to do more worthwhile things in life than they can without it, then health work is a far broader endeavour than the official activities of the NHS. Once it is seen and acknowledged that autonomy is the basic constituent of health care activity then the Fortress must collapse, and those inside it will be left to compete with all other health workers for the resources to create more autonomy in the world.

Instrumental Need with the End of Increasing Autonomy

Given the above purpose it follows that the way to understand need in relation to health work is, always, **as a gap which must be filled if there is to be more autonomy**. The benefit or supply definition is therefore quite inadequate to explain health need, as is any definition of need which assumes man-made limits on what can be needed. The only definitions of need which make sense beyond the Fortress are instrumental need defined by the individual who is seeking more health, and normative need where the expert health worker is genuinely attempting to create further autonomy. If these two understandings clash then the way to resolve them is to assume that the individual has a clearer view of what will empower her than the health worker unless there are very good reasons to doubt this.[128] In any case, given the basic purpose of health care, any proposal to go against a person's reasoned views must always be very carefully thought through since this is a *prima facie* undermining of autonomy. If after this the matter remains in doubt it will be necessary to ask, and clarify in the fullest practical detail, which of the range of options open will create more autonomy.[129]

Where groups of people are concerned, surveys of their health needs should not be restricted to what the inhabitants of the Fortress are interested in or can supply. If this restriction applies then 'needs-assessment surveys' can be nothing more than self-fulfilling prophecies which must inevitably reinforce the fortifications, and which – if they increase the autonomy of the surveyed set at all – do so only incidentally.

Taking Quality Seriously

When knowledge of the basic purpose of health care is coupled with the findings of the investigation into the meaning of quality outside the Fortress, it becomes even more apparent – unless reason is brazenly ignored – that the expertise of all people must be taken into account when planning health services. Once quality is taken seriously, once it is recognised that fashionable business terminology corrupts the meaning of an important ideal, then the requirement to engage all those with an interest in the NHS and its organisation is overwhelming. No doubt it will be difficult, no doubt a great deal of education will have to be done in order to bring people into a position where they can debate the full range of issues, and no doubt the effort will be financially costly – but the human benefits would be immense. It is, of course, not possible to predict accurately what people will say about such choices as – 'would you prefer to spend the nation's wealth to ensure that everyone who wants one has a home, or would you prefer to maintain the present level of spending on pharmaceuticals and new technology?' – but it is surely important that we are asked, and not least because both policies may add to the autonomy of the nation's people, and yet at the moment only one is given the opportunity to do so.

Less grandly, at the level of hospital wards and the everyday delivery of medical services, if quality is taken seriously then people must be consulted about what they want and about what they think, and they must be asked in an open way – not with questions that prejudge the merit of the continued existence of Fortress NHS. Thus the old people whom the managers are considering relocating must be asked what they think; first because not to do so is already to subvert their autonomy, second because unless this is done their hierarchy of instrumental needs will not be known, and thirdly because not to do so is to ignore their expertise and competence as human beings. They will know better than anyone what makes them feel safe, what makes them happy, and what continues to challenge them. The managers must recognise that the extent to which the old people's views are overlooked is the extent to which real quality will be lost.

The philosophical analysis of quality, coupled with a philosophical understanding of the nature of health, reveals one further significant insight. This is that quality, as it is perceived in the present generally purposeless Fortress, is associated only with **function**, and not with **moral function**. However, once it is understood that working for health is a moral endeavour,[127] quality in health care must be associated with **moral function**.

The importance of this distinction can be demonstrated by reference to the brief example of the torturer (see p. 52). As things stand – in an NHS which does not have a clear definition of health and purpose – if the torturer was employed by the NHS she could quite validly be described as a quality torturer so long as her work was deemed fit for the purpose required within the Fortress. It would not be theoretically possible to object to this description since there would be no countermanding theory of health to bring into play. However, if work for health is seen as essentially an endeavour to enable fulfilling potential, and if quality in health care is correctly seen as part of this idea rather than as a commercial strategy, it becomes quite wrong to describe the work of the torturer as quality. On this view quality in health care and quality in torturing rightly become worlds apart.

Equalising to Create Autonomy without the Fortress

If egalitarianism is considered to be an important principle of health, and this notion is certainly consistent with the view that autonomy in the most basic sense is important to all people equally, then – since it only has real meaning without the Fortress – policies based on it must be carried out in the interest of health in society in general. Quite simply, if there are people in society with very low levels of autonomy, and if it is possible to distribute resources to enable them to have more autonomy, then their cases should be considered as the first priority. Their impoverished levels of autonomy should not only come up for attention when they fall sick – or even when they fall under the view of other 'caring Fortresses' in Britain. Rather, the whole structure of society should be such that all people are ensured a basic level of autonomy to enable them to move in life without constant pressure and anxiety. Clearly many British people are currently not enabled in this way so, if improving their health is to be considered as a serious priority, policies should be proposed (and should then be subject to open and informed discussion) to reallocate resources from richer systems (at least to the point suggested elsewhere[65,67]).

This recommendation follows simply from the premises that autonomy is basic to health, and that it is important for all people. Naturally, however, there are very many objections to such an idea – indeed any which have ever been argued against any form of egalitarianism might be set against it.[63,64] One possible objection seems particularly weighty. This is that some people – the severely mentally handicapped, the sick who need very expensive treatments to remain alive, and people with profound physical disabilities – can often never achieve even the basic level of autonomy which the system of welfare suggested here would set. Even to try to raise levels of autonomy in order to 'equalise' this unfortunate group of people the rest of us would have to undergo such hardship as to make the 'equalising' untenable. However, although this point of view is clearly substantial, it is not obviously correct.

Firstly it is not the case that a policy of equalising for health must necessarily seek to bring everyone up to the 'same level' of welfare. What it would do would be to seek to bring out those potentials in the severely unautonomous which they would find fulfilling. For some this would indeed be very expensive, but efforts need not be blindly heroic – realistic goals would be enough.[67] And not to try in lives which might have more autonomy with more investment (choosing instead to invest in more fortunate lives) is to say that some people are naturally more important than others. In many respects of course this is true, some people contribute a lot to society and others simply consume. But the price of drawing the conclusion from this that therefore the 'best' people should have autonomy creating services at the expense of the 'mere consumers' is enormous. This is not the place to reflect more deeply on political philosophy (though such reflection is sooner or later inevitable when one is considering the provision of health care). All that it is necessary to say at this point is that such a policy – where autonomy for one person is thought more important than autonomy for another – inevitably results in activities towards the underprivileged which cannot fittingly be called health care activities.

The question of whether supporting the most able people actually results in greater benefits for the weakest is a constant subject of political and economic debate, and is beyond the remit of this account.

Preventing the Sacrifice of Autonomy without the Fortress

Towards the end of the penultimate paper in this series it was suggested that one logical consequence of thinking of cost as sacrifice was the question: **which sorts of human effort will produce the greatest autonomy at least cost in loss of autonomy to others?** It was argued that this question could be asked properly only if it is accepted that the NHS version of 'work for health' is limited, and confined within Fortress walls. If this view is accepted it can form a central element of the framework of a reformed health service. Under this guiding idea plans might be drawn up to design a system of services to create autonomy. On the face of it this seems to be an impossible task both in practice and theory: the Fortress is very strong and it is not the only one in Britain, and even theoretically it is difficult to see how to begin with such an enormous, general project.

Ways in which to achieve practical change are, by and large, beyond my expertise. Certainly changes would not be easy – at the very least it would require far more radical developments than Bevan and other Ministers of the Labour Government of the 1940s were able to bring about. But it would be too much to say that it is impossible.

The theoretical task is at least slightly easier than the practical. A full defence of the foundations of services designed to create autonomy must be left for a later work, but the following points at least are already clear. If the basic cost of doing something is the best of whatever else could have been done instead, and if the basic purpose of health care activity is the increase of people's control over their worlds, then the cost of any particular health work activity is the greatest increase in autonomy that could have been had instead. Now clearly the notion of autonomy could be further categorised into various 'types of control' – and would have to be if difficult judgements were to be made about cost conceived in this way – but this is not the present purpose. Instead, the question is this: in general is it in principle better to supply a little more of something to a person when that person already has a lot of it, or is it better to supply a little more of something to a person who has only a little to begin with? In practice, the answer must be that it depends upon specific circumstances, what the type of control is, and what further sorts of autonomy the additional autonomy will release. But in theory it is reasonable to assume that the latter alternative should be preferred – that is, that the weakest should have their levels of control raised first, so as to enable them to live more fulfilling lives*. A policy of equalising without the Fortress must concentrate the nation's resources first on the weak rather than on the economically productive (and so, for instance, might in practice demand a reduction in the wages of well-paid medical consultants in order to provide better support for educationally sub-normal infants). And even if the policy would not directly redistribute money from the pockets of one group into the hands of another, it would mean that only when sufficient services to enable the least autonomous people to have meaningful control over their lives are in place should the nation's resources be spent on providing for the most autonomous people (who are usually very well equipped to pay for what they want anyway).

This conclusion is in direct opposition to the developing views of many health economists (even though it is quite compatible with most of their logic), and is certainly opposed to those of the American right wing. However, if a person's life has no meaning then the addition of only a little life purpose is priceless. And where there is little autonomy in the first place it might be argued that additional autonomy for that person is far more precious than the freedom of a wealthy family to purchase a new dishwasher or an extra car. This notion is also consistent with the economic theory of marginal utility and, where nations are wealthy and are familiar with the notion of **luxury**, the view has obvious moral merit.

Used in line with the strongest parts of the other health service principles such a policy is certainly equalising (whereas the present policies of the NHS are usually not), it insists that some very basic needs (or gaps) should be filled before any others are, and not only is it designed to improve people's 'quality of life' according to the common meaning of the phrase, but also it should bring more people into the position where they can become involved in setting true quality standards for public services.

---

* Thus the logic of economics is restricted by the morality of welfare.

Planning

All this, even at the abstract level outlined so far, quite obviously requires a plan. Vision and the formulation of detailed plans and policies are rare in present times, and appear to be virtually extinct in the NHS. Rather than think seriously about what services are most important, and most certainly in preference to challenging established commercial interests,[109] current 'health service planning' amounts to little more than attempting to reduce expenditure by enforcing cuts in the most vulnerable areas, and hoping that by running health services based on inaccurate models of business, things will become more efficient (even though, as has been seen, no-one is sure even about what 'becoming more efficient' means). A social plan, on the other hand, requires deep thought by many people with a range of expertise and interests.

It is possible for a government safely in office to do pretty well anything it wishes. If a plan based on the notions explained above were to be formulated then inevitably great changes would ensue (if our reigning political masters were brave and honest enough) – unless those presently in charge of the Fortress could demonstrate that in every case their endeavours were least costly of autonomy. In order to have the plan discussed democratically it would be necessary to invest resources in a massive programme of public education and debate – which in itself could not be debated prior to its enactment. However, so long as the intent of the programme was ultimately to seek the informed views of the population then its initially non-democratic nature could be justified. Certainly, over the past decade and a half the government has concentrated enormous resources on very simplistic (and often very dubious) 'education campaigns'[130,131,132] without any such democratic intention, and has apparently felt justified in its actions.

Objections

Naturally this proposed basis for the reform of health services is open to a huge selection of objections, only a few of which can even be mentioned here. However, it is important to discuss possible responses to two of the strongest.

1. The Framework Cannot Cope with Hard Choices

The basic framework outlined above has not been developed to the extent where it could be used to justify the hard judgements which decision-making in scarcity (which would remain) require – it is too vague. It would not, for instance, be of any help in a case where a decision had to be made over which of a number of people should receive the only treatment available (although it would supply a basic structure within which a conversation about the problem could take place). However, although the general framework outlined in these papers does not give answers to the 'hard choices', many other methods already exist to assist decision-making in tricky cases.[126,133,134] None is absolute and none is particularly precise, but to look for a highly accurate decision-making implement for the complex judgements in life is to run after a mirage.

But this is not the present point. The basic point is that before any such hard choices can be rationally addressed it is essential that a basic, coherent system is in place – ideally one which ensures the chance of a fulfilling life for each and every member of a population. Then, and only then, can the 'hard choices' be openly addressed. Once such a civilised system is in place then further precision might be sought. For instance, different general **types** of decision might be identified. For instance, categories might be constructed which would enable the formulation of **general policy decisions** (such as deciding what the set of 'central autonomy services' ought to be, or in times of plenty what extra enabling facilities ought to be generally provided); decisions which might be made through **open democracy**; decisions which would be the province of those **in charge of administering** whatever level and sorts of services exist; decisions made by **individual helpers** about their priorities; and decisions which should be made through **discussion** between all interested individuals and groups. Controversy would be inevitable, as always, but at least debate would be carried out in the knowledge that basic autonomy-creating services were available for everyone.

At the moment there is a sort of madness abroad. It is as if we must always take decisions in a back-to-front fashion. Many of the hard choices of health care are simply the result of the lack of planning, and derive from the fact that the financial profit motive has led companies to fund expensive research which produces scarce therapies. The inverted logic is that because a beneficial service has come into being, and a form of therapy is therefore possible, it simply must be undertaken. So long as it has benefit (and it must if there are 'hard choices' to be made about who gets it, so the reasoning goes) then we cannot possibly contemplate not continuing with it (indeed we must have more if we possibly can). The simple-minded tendency is to see that some benefit is possible, and so also to see the therapy as clearly desirable – and thus the perpetuation of the craziness is ensured.

At the moment, any hard choices which have somehow been brought about through human design can be seen as artificial choices to which there are only artificial answers. To state an extreme example, where a decision has to be reached over which of two obese people should receive some form of dietary therapy first, and there are people starving in the world, then any deliberation about the merits of the two potential patients is obviously contrived.

Of course, this is not only a philosophical conclusion. It is shared by many thoughtful commentators on the NHS, as the following extract from a newspaper leader article shows. It is merely to be hoped that the philosophical perspective outlined in this collection of papers will further strengthen constructive criticism of the Fortress:

The health service has become 'too bureaucratic' under the Government's restructuring. Who says so? No, not the new Labour health spokesman sharpening up his rhetoric in preparation for party conference time, but the Government's junior health minister, Lady Cumberledge, a minister with wide experience of the NHS. She was explaining on Friday the Government's decision to seek ways of making it easier for patients to be treated at hospitals of their choice. Contrary to ministerial claims, the present structure blocks this through hospitals having to restrict their treatment to patients from local health authorities with which they have contracts. Some leeway is provided through a special procedure (known as extra-contractual referrals), but over 10 000 patients were refused treatment last year because their local health authority had run out of money for these referrals.

The process has become a labyrinthine paper chase, which has diverted a large amount of managerial energy and effort. For the mediocre and those steeped in administration rather than management, this has been a welcome diversion. Chasing bills and monitoring contracts is far easier than thinking strategically about how to deliver health services. Ministers are right to step in, but they were warned from the beginning – in these columns and by other critics – of the paper avalanche they were creating. Now, ironically, ministers are talking of allowing family doctors the freedom to refer patients to wherever they wish within a prescribed budget. This is where we came in four years ago.

The paradoxes do not stop there. Belatedly, ministers have also recognised the danger of allowing hospitals and community services to opt out together. A change was signalled last week in a letter inviting bids for the fourth and last big wave of opted out NHS trusts due to come into operation in 1994. The new guidance says community health services must in general be run separately from hospitals. The reason is not hard to fathom. The Royal London is only one of several London teaching hospitals that have raided their community services budget to maintain hospital services. Historically, hospitals have always been more powerful than community health services. The last 40 years has seen successive governments struggle to redistribute resources from ever burgeoning hospital budgets, which only account for one out of 10 patients using the NHS, to preventive and primary health care provided by community services. The new structure has only made this more acute, according to a letter last week from nine professional organisations and three royal colleges which suggests primary care has become even more fragmented. It urges ministers to create a more unified approach.

All of which makes sense, but one warning is needed, Ministers have become obsessed with structure. They continued to fiddle around as though with one final adjustment, the model will have been perfected. It won't be. The model does need radical pruning, but Ministers need to remember the purpose of the NHS is its services – not its structure. Separating hospital and community services is sensible, but it should not be an iron rule. Some parts of the country have begun to experiment with innovative community support services and post-operative rehabilitation units closer to people's homes. They should be allowed to continue.[135]

2. The Framework Leads Ultimately to the Use of a Version of the QALY

Since part of the inspiration of the QALY was an implicit theory of health which emphasised people's ability to do fulfilling things, there are naturally some similarities between the framework and the health economists' measure. However, the differences are far more significant.

Firstly the QALY is not intended as a basis for the reform of the NHS, only as a tool to be used within the Fortress. Secondly, its methodology is dubious to say the least. Thirdly, its use tends to discriminate against the weakest people – in particular the use of the QALY in cases where severely mentally and physically handicapped people require scarce medical resources must always mean that the 'able bodied' will receive the resources first (unless it is known that they have only a very short time left to live). Fourthly, it encourages neither education nor the involvement of 'the subjects of care' since the method of calculation is based on prior surveys. And fifthly it has been shown elsewhere how practical systems of deliberation – of a more precise nature than the general framework – can **incorporate** the QALY as one part of a more extensive decision-making process.[126]

CONCLUSION

Constructing A Genuine Health Service: A Practical and Philosophical Challenge

In order to develop a philosophy of health of relevance to health professionals it is necessary to try to learn as much as possible about the reality of health work. In so doing it quickly becomes obvious that the sorts of speculations which might hold water in a philosophy seminar will appear naive to those working to survive, and to succeed where they can, in far less rational environments. This dissonance between calm intellectual analysis and the practical turmoil of human politics poses a considerable challenge for anyone who wishes to think deeply about, and ultimately suggest solutions to the problems faced by the NHS.

The Need for a Plan

Essentially the challenge is this. The health service makes very little philosophical sense, so attempting to improve policy philosophically is like trying to mix oil and water – yet further politically inspired changes cannot possibly succeed in making the service more coherent either. Therefore, the only way to a more sensible service is to work out a general plan removed from daily struggles, and then seek agreement to it. Without a plan there can only be more of the same – more power games, more manipulation of the system for incompatible and often selfish ends, and more nonsense written to try to justify the philosophically indefensible. But of course even a generally reasoned programme for major reform is unlikely to be properly understood by those within the health service either because they will see their world through different eyes, or because they will not wish for reforms which will interfere with behaviours which are producing success on their terms. So the situation facing those who would like to see more rational reform is not encouraging, and may even be desperate. But it is not hopeless.

The Way in

The secret of preventing change in any system is to stop up all channels through which protests might meaningfully be heard. The NHS has managed to achieve this in practice through a host of direct methods.[2,3,5,51] Its perimeter defences and outer walls are as robust as ever. Indeed it is difficult to overestimate the practical power of those who benefit most from the Fortress – and impossible not to continue to be shocked by the often quite brazen corruption encountered when examining its practices first hand. And of course naked exploitation is not all there is. There is much subtlety too. Perhaps the most devious effort so far rests with the organisation's use of words. If the only form of expression permitted within the Fortress is a polluted and enfeebled pseudo-technical language then, it is assumed, this may be enough on its own to frustrate reform through Reason. But to seek to prohibit free speech and intelligent debate is never a sign of real strength.

Anyone who builds a Fortress does so because he is afraid of something. Fortresses are not particularly pleasant places to live – they confine their inhabitants and restrict their movements, they are nervous and conservative places, and they are very incestuous. When those outside the Fortress see the occupants building fresh fortifications they might well be led to despair, but they might also – and with justification – take the fresh construction works as a symptom of internal decay. The frantic management-speak and 'advertising front' of the 1990s is not the mark of a company which knows where it is going – far from it. The verbose veneer is compelling evidence of a fundamental loss of confidence.

The way to dismantle the Fortress is not to hurl stones at it from the outside, but to show it up for what it is. It is by no means entirely bad – very many of its members do not realise that they are trapped within it, and offer devoted and selfless help to people in difficulty, but such people are rarely the Fortress chiefs. It is those at the top, those who know most about the Fortress who are responsible for its continuation, and their guilt is no small matter.

Of course even the most powerful members of Fortress NHS cannot be blamed for the ills of the world, or for the fact that many people in Britain (never mind the rest of the planet) live unhappy, underdeveloped and unfulfilled lives. The responsibility for this sad state of affairs cannot be laid at their door alone. The lack of comprehensive welfare facilities is not only the fault of those who control medical services. However, it is hard to deny that the status of medicine (and the myths which surround it in Britain) constantly detracts attention from more general human need,[136] seems to offer a safety net to excuse the Government from directing more funds to general welfare schemes, and above all stands on very fragile conceptual ground.

The directors of Fortress NHS undoubtedly contribute to the perpetuation of a poorer world. They control vast amounts of the nation's wealth (not a little of which finds its way into their own pockets), and they are responsible for directing that wealth down certain avenues before others without proper justification. Therefore, every time they engage in their games, every time they decide that they must have the latest gadget in preference to a more enabling alternative, every time they organise a conference to discuss words and policies already in use but not understood, and every time they drive to their fortress past people with downturned faces walking shabby streets, they are guilty of the most fundamental negligence: the witting sacrifice of autonomy. The most guilty are the ones who know best what they are doing, the ones who know that there is no coherent set of purposes in the NHS, but are as clear as day about their own. But whenever they go to a board meeting and go along with what they know to be theatre when they could be using their intelligence to ask unsettling questions, or to direct resources to the most needy people outside the Fortress as well as in – then they are culpable. And the saddest fact of all is that they know it. Whatever the personal pressures, whatever the demands of the system, to go knowingly along with the show when better things might be done is the most basic dereliction of a human duty to other people.

Dialogue Four

Escape from the Fortress

Tempers are becoming frayed in the boardroom. Despite Melanie's advice, the philosopher has been called to explain his failure. The original committee members are all present, and it is too hot in the room.

Dr Graham: (to Donald Arthur) . . . the absence of alternative suggestions – despite what I take to be your best efforts – surely means that the only option now open is to close the ward.

Donald Arthur: I think it does look that way. As you say, 'thinking time' is limited just like everything else in this hospital. However, that is not to say that more thinking time would not produce a better option . . .

Dr Graham: I hope that's not a veiled request for an extension to the working party Donald. I think it's quite clear that more thinking will only produce more confusion. Before our ethicist friend became involved the problem was difficult – now it seems to be almost insoluble. If you have any more time we may well end up entirely paralysed. Enough's enough.

Melanie Smith: I don't think that's right. I too am disappointed that we do not have a clear answer for you, but I don't think that our failure to come up with clear suggestions after only a few days is surprising. Wouldn't it have been more surprising if we had?

Dr Graham: I don't see why. Most committees produce answers on tight deadlines these days. Why should yours be an exception?

Philosopher: May I answer that question?

Dr Graham: Please be brief. You have already had a chance to make your case.

Philosopher: Yes I know, but I think none of you listened to me.

Peter Walker: Of course we did. And we took minutes.

Philosopher: Of course you heard my words but I do not believe – in fact I'm positive – that you did not fully comprehend my meaning. None of you – not even Melanie – understand what I'm trying to say.

Melanie: (a little hurt) Oh.

Philosopher: For example, Melanie is optimistic enough to think that we could come up with a better plan if we had spent longer working on it – and perhaps if more of the working party had managed to attend more meetings. And you, Dr Graham, think that I've shown the problem to be **almost** insoluble. But you are both quite wrong. In truth your problem is at once soluble and insoluble. To solve it we do not need any more time, yet if we had all the time in the world we could never solve it under present circumstances.

Melanie: Stop talking in riddles. And stop showing off.

Philosopher: (*firmly*) What I mean is that you have very many *ad hoc* solutions available to you – you can close the ward, you can increase the car parking charges, you can sell capital, you can cut staff, you can charge £30 a night for a bed if you like. All these are solutions within the 'system' you have inherited. There is, however, ultimately little to choose between them since each solution will create further dilemmas of the same basic type. My objection to this approach – I think some of you call it 'fire-fighting' – is very simple: **solutions derived *ad hoc*, from an irrational system, are not meaningful solutions because you cannot give a consistent account of why one is better than another**. And the reason you cannot give a consistent account of why one solution is to be preferred over another is because you do not have a clear view of the purpose of your 'system'.

This is why I, as a trained philosopher, cannot solve the problem in your system. You do not apply your logic consistently, most decisions are not justified theoretically – nor do you have the means to justify them even if you wished to do so – and what's more your 'system' is driven continually by commercial forces external to it. To me – among other images – the NHS looks like a cork bobbing helplessly in the unpredictable current of a great river.

Of course, this doesn't mean that your problem is permanently insoluble. Far from it. It is perfectly and rationally soluble within alternative systems. Indeed, in some systems it would never have arisen in the first place.

Melanie: But we can't change the system. We have no choice but to work within it.

Philosopher: Then you will never find the solutions you think you are looking for. (*There is silence, for a moment*). Let me show you what I mean. And then – before you dismiss me as incurably idealistic – let me explain a little of a philosophy of health which could create a more rational health service. In other words, let me show you how you might invent a different health system.

Donald Arthur: Five minutes, then we must close the meeting.

Philosopher: Let's say that you have recently been able to supply a very expensive treatment, but only to a select few people. This treatment will place a financial burden on your hospital, but if you help pioneer the treatment the company who has invented it will offer future supplies at 20% less than standard cost. If the treatment comes to be used widely then your hospital will stand to make substantial savings. What is more, the chances are that the treatment will help those who receive it to live pain-free lives for several years longer than they would otherwise be expected to.

From your point of view, from within your 'system', it makes sense to take up the offer since it looks like you will have a chance to 'expand' or 'develop'. You don't know precisely what shape this 'expansion' will take, but nevertheless it looks like a good thing. Now, my point is that not only does this decision not have the benefit of a view of what progress is, but also that by taking it you prevent other patients, with other complaints, in your hospital from experiencing similar expansion, what's more, you make the decision in competition with other hospitals who are supposed to be part of a wider whole (and so in competition with claims of patients elsewhere), and also in competition with alternative ways of spending public money to make lives better – not in hospitals. You do this even when you appeal to charity for support. That money for the CAT scanner, that emotive fund-raising for the children's ward, that 'Silver Heart' campaign – it all means that other welfare initiatives cannot take place as a result.

You will say to me that this is simply the way life is; that hospitals do not have bottomless budgets, that you are bound to think first of your own hospital, that your use of charitable support is as good as anyone else's, that industries are organised so as to produce goods which people find of benefit – and which make the company a profit – that the Government provides cash in parcels marked 'health', 'social services', 'transport', 'housing' etc., and that you cannot change this and so should try to get as much of whatever is going as possible. If this doesn't make sense overall it is not your problem, and even if you were to take it on as a problem there is nothing you could do to change things. You will say to me that I am looking for rationality which does not – cannot possibly – exist, that the world is uncertain, that we must make the most of it, that we must take chances we hope will turn out well, that more than this is asking too much of human beings.

But I can reply with equal fervour, for what seems like pragmatism to you looks like fatalism to me. I will say to you that there is nothing you can tell me about 'the real world'. I live here too, and I know what has to be done to get by in it. I also know how powerless I am to change any of it, and I know how it can seem obvious that one must accept the world the way it is. But I cannot accept what you seem to. I cannot accept it in practice and I cannot accept it in theory – even if there's nothing, apparently, that I can do about it.

What is it like outside this hospital? What are people's lives like? You know as much as I do. You know how many people around here have no work to do, you know the dereliction, you know what dreary houses lie around this compound. You also know something of the people's ignorance, and of what they can hope for, and if you are honest you know that more often than not it is not very much. The children around here have children of their own to give them something to do, or to give them a house of their own. If they get a job they are lucky, and if they find something to challenge them they are far luckier still. They get old early, they can be weary of the world when they are six, and they do not grow – only older.

Not everyone has such a life, and not everyone who lives in this district is submerged in so much dullness. But a lot are. Little is spent on them, little is done for them – unless they break the law or unless they become sick or injured. When they do, and especially if they are sick, then they may have a fortune spent on them. They may, if they are 'lucky', have expensive and extensive diagnostic tests, prolonged therapy and rehabilitation (again if they are lucky) and then – if they survive and recover – they go back to the dullness. Schemes designed to add meaning to people's lives already exist: for example care in the community **can** mean efforts to integrate people with difficult lives so as to give them more purpose; in some hospitals there are genuine attempts to involve parents in the care of their children whilst on the wards; and for some in health promotion and public health the priority is not always less morbidity – the goal can, sometimes, be more involvement in social life.

But such projects are little more than candles in the dark. There is no overall reason for most current health work which can be sustained theoretically. If people are worth attention when they are sick why are they not worth attention when their lives are unfulfilled? Unless the treatment of sickness is to lead to more fulfilment what is the point of it?

And this is where I believe I have an answer – and the basis for a new system – and where you do not. I have a view about why it is worth intervening in people's lives – actually in their lives rather than in a way which will impact on morbidity and mortality statistics. I have a purposive theory of health work whereas you have a historically conditioned reaction to disease.

Let me explain a little more. The health system I would develop instead of your medically dominated one draws on a theory that **health is the foundations for achievement**. This theory, although apparently very straightforward, has a fairly complicated philosophical underpinning which there is no time to explain to you. (*He* *points to a pile of books at his side*). Donald, you can read about it in these books if you want the detail. In brief summary it looks like this:

The basic idea is that if you want to know whether a person is healthy or not you do not necessarily have to ask a doctor, rather you need to examine the state of the 'platform' on which the person in question is able to move, or perform in life. The stronger the platform the healthier the person. So, if a person has a fulfilling job, a warm and safe home, good and varied information, the skills to assimilate and make sense of this information, and also is aware that all other people need strong platforms on which to live, then he or she can be said to be healthy. Even if the person who has these foundations for achievement is diseased then she still may have a high degree of health. And if the disease is not interfering in her life – if for instance she has optimal movement on her stage but also has a disease – then she may have **maximum health** for her, **and** be diseased.

Of course, it is often the case that to suffer a disease or injury is to have **restricted** movement in life, and that to work to eliminate such problems is properly work for health. But it is not true that work against disease is therefore **central** to work for health. What is **central** to work for health depends upon the condition of an individual's platform for autonomy, and is whatever problem is presenting the biggest obstacle to a person's worthwhile life movement at a particular time.

On this theory of health the first question is not: how can I control health service costs? or how can I decide which anti-disease measure to invest in? but, how can I ensure the maximum possible movement in life for everyone? Which is to say: how can I work to ensure the strongest platform for everyone and so create the most, and most widespread, health? On this theory of health the question which confronts you as: 'should I close the ward?' could not be asked. Instead, you would ask 'within the population supported by the health service which parts of which platforms need the most urgent attention?' Or to put this another way you would ask: 'which people have least movement in life, who has least autonomy, and how can I direct health services to support them?'.

This approach is very different from the one you have. For a start, it is consistently positive – it looks to what might be in the future as its *raison d'être*, not simply at present disease. It has a clear purpose – to raise levels of autonomy for everyone, and to focus first on those who have least – certainly up to the point where everyone possesses the basic foundations for achievement or, if this is not possible, where everyone has sufficient support to ensure a meaningful life. It is not orchestrated by outside interests, and what counts as success in this system is clear – and this success is certainly far easier to assess than it is in your system. All that is necessary to evaluate work for health on my system is to set clear standards for the foundations (and in part they set themselves because they must be sufficient to allow creative movement in the lives of individuals) and to check that these are achieved. Rather than design Heath Robinson measures of 'well-being', 'health status', and 'health gain' – and rather than demean the human condition by thinking of health only as a decrease in morbidity – it is possible to measure health on this theory by checking whether people have homes, by asking what they can do, by finding out what they know, what time they have, what demands work makes on them, what they have learnt at work, what the opportunities for further learning at work are, and so on.

It can be done, and it is not difficult in principle. Only it will never happen if people like you adopt vacuous theories of health by default. Let me be crystal clear: medical work may be a part of health work, but also may not be. Everything depends upon whether the work adds to a person's movement in life. If it is not intended to so add then it is not health work. Other work, other forms of provision are equally part of health work, and often can be of much greater importance than medicine. Again, it depends on the freedom in life each creates.

On this theory of health you must examine the elderly people's foundations for achievement and build them up where they are weakest. If this leads you to close the ward then so be it, but at least you will have a theoretical reason for doing so. I think you should approach the problem as a 'foundational' one, even if others are not yet doing so. Why not build upon all the positive things which are happening here? Why not take the initiatives inspired by a broader notion of health taken in this very hospital, express and justify them theoretically, build on them and try to develop many more of the same? Why not listen to the nurses who say they need more time to talk to patients? Why not regard this as proper health work – real therapy? Why don't you ask the patients what they value the most? Don't use closed questionnaires with loaded questions – just ask them. Why not ask the junior doctors how they would improve things? Why must you always go along with the crowd? What's so intimidating about questioning the questionable? Why not examine prescribing habits and drug budgets, not with a view to cost reduction but with an open mind? Why not ask – do we need all this? Why not ask – are there alternatives? For if you do you will surely find that there are, and you may be surprised at what so-called 'fringe' therapies can achieve. Why not – in short – open yourselves up to change, and open up your fortress to debate? Real debate with no questions barred. You could begin a revolution – a revolution in thinking required to have a real health service rather than an imperial medical army. If you did you would not find a true solution immediately – indeed solutions might seem further away at first, but you would be part of a move towards the possibility of true solutions.

You see there are answers, but within the present system they are not theoretically sustainable. If I were to offer you an answer on your terms then I would truly have failed. But if I offer you a way out, and you don't even try it, then the failure is yours.

Ending One

Dr Graham: I have never heard so much nonsense in my life. Mr Ethicist, you are quite useless. You read, you get paid to think, and then you rant. But none of it is any help to us. We have to make a decision and we cannot change the world. We will close the ward, the old people will survive or they will die – much as they would have done on the ward. There will be no controversy, we will be credible, we will try to improve our services whenever we can – and the hospital will go on.

We do not need you. You have nothing to offer us.

Ending Two

Melanie: Before Dr Graham closes the meeting – before we decide on the ward closure – I'd like to respond personally to what we have heard, and to what some of us have read this week.

I have very mixed feelings. I can see the logic of the philosopher's arguments – at least I can see some of it – and I think his sentiments are genuine. I can also see that what he says about us not ultimately solving anything is important. But what worries me is that the alternative is not clear. What would the 'new NHS' look like? What would it cost? What would it do? What would it not do? Who would manage it? How would the medical profession feel about taking a lesser role? Wouldn't such an upheaval be dangerous?

Philosopher: Yes, of course it would be dangerous, but so is the present system for all the reasons I've explained earlier.

As for your other points, there is plenty of foundational literature available on 'the new NHS' already. There are many theories of health, some of which have already been highly developed and argued (far more than any official health service theory). What is required now is the will to apply such theories to reform the health service. Given such a will your practical questions could be answered, and would be answered in a theoretically consistent fashion. Given the will the present NHS could be demolished – not overnight but steadily and with a clear end in sight. In its place there could be a service which has principles with substance – a service designed to equalise, to provide the means towards fulfilled lives for all, and to do so democratically. A rational service is possible, I don't think that's in question. The real question is: are there enough brave people in the Fortress to give real reform a chance? Are there enough people even **aware** of the Fortress? There is no escape unless you know your prison.

Appendix One

The Beveridge Report and the Role of a Health Service

Assumption B. Comprehensive Health and Rehabilitation Services

426. The second of the three assumptions has two sides to it. It covers a national health service for prevention and for cure of disease and disability by medical treatment; it covers rehabilitation and fitting for employment by treatment which will be both medical and post-medical. Administratively, realisation of Assumption B on its two sides involves action both by the departments concerned with health and by the Minister of Labour and National Service. Exactly where the line should be drawn between the responsibilities of these Departments cannot, and need not, be settled now. For the purpose of the present Report, the two sides are combined under one head, avoiding the need to distinguish accurately at this stage between medical and post-medical work. The case for regarding Assumption B as necessary for a satisfactory system of social security needs little emphasis. It is a logical corollary to the payment of high benefits in disability that determined efforts should be made by the State to reduce the number of cases for which benefit is needed. It is a logical corollary to the receipt of high benefits in disability that the individual should recognise the duty to be well and to co-operate in all steps which may lead to diagnosis of disease in early stages when it can be prevented. Disease and accidents must be paid for in any case, in lessened power of production and in idleness, if not directly by insurance benefits. One of the reasons why it is preferable to pay for disease and accident openly and directly in the form of insurance benefits, rather than indirectly, is that this emphasises the cost and should give a stimulus to prevention. As to the methods of realising Assumption B, the main problems naturally arise under the first head of medical treatment. Rehabilitation is a new field of remedial activity with great possibilities, but requiring expenditure of a different order of magnitude from that involved in the medical treatment of the nation.

427. The first part of Assumption B is that a comprehensive national health service will ensure that for every citizen there is available whatever medical treatment he requires, in whatever form he requires it, domiciliary or institutional, general, specialist or consultant, and will ensure also the provision of dental, ophthalmic and surgical appliances, nursing and midwifery and rehabilitation after accidents. Whether or not payment towards the cost of the health service is included in the social insurance contribution, the service itself should:

1. be organised, not only by the Ministry concerned with social insurance, but by Departments, responsible for the health of the people and for positive and preventive as well as curative measures;
2. be provided where needed without contribution conditions in any individual case.

Restoration of a sick person to health is a duty of the State and the sick person, prior to any other consideration. The assumption made here is in accord with the definition of the objects of medical service as proposed in the Draft Interim Report of the Medical Planning Commission of the British Medical Association:

a) to provide a system of medical service directed towards the achievement of positive health, of the prevention of disease, and the relief of sickness;
b) to render available to every individual all necessary medical services, general and specialist, and both domiciliary and institutional.

From: Beveridge, W. (Chairman) (1942) *Report on Social Insurance and Allied Services*, Cmd 6404, London: HMSO, paras 426–7, reproduced by permission.

Appendix Two

The 1944 White Paper

The record of this country in its health and medical services is a good one. The resistance of people to the wear and tear of four years of a second world war bears testimony to it. Achievements before the war – in lower mortality rates, in the gradual decline of many of the more serious diseases, in safer motherhood and healthier childhood, and generally in the prospect of a longer and healthier life – all substantiate it. There is no question of having to abandon bad services and to start afresh. Reform in this field is not a matter of making good what is bad, but of making better what is good already.

The present system has its origins deep in the history of the country's social services. Broadly, it is the product of the last hundred years, though some of its elements go much farther back. But most of the impetus has been gathered in the last generation or two, and it was left to the present century to develop most of the personal health services as they are now known . . ..

The main reason for change is that the Government believe that, at this stage of social development, the care of personal health should be put on a new footing and be made available to everybody as a publicly sponsored service. Just as people are accustomed to look to public organisation for essential facilities like a clean and safe water supply or good highways, accepting these as things which the community combines to provide for the benefit of the individual without distinction of section or group, so they should now be able to look for proper facilities for the care of their personal health to a publicly organised service available to all who want to use it – a service for which all would be paying as taxpayers and ratepayers and contributors to some national scheme of social insurance.

In spite of the substantial progress of many years and the many good services built up under public authority and by voluntary and private effort, it is still not true to say that everyone can get all the kinds of medical and hospital service which he or she may require. Whether people can do so still depends too much upon circumstances, upon where they happen to live or work, to what group (e.g. of age, or vocation) they happen to belong, or what happens to be the matter with them. Nor is the care of health yet wholly divorced from ability to pay for it, although great progress has already been made in eliminating the financial barrier to obtaining most of the essential services. There is not yet, in short, a comprehensive cover for health provided for all people alike. That is what it is now the Government's intention to provide.

To take one very important example, the first-line care of health for everyone requires a personal doctor or a family doctor, a general medical practitioner available for consultation on all problems of health and sickness. At present, the National Health Service Insurance scheme makes this provision for a large number of people; but it does not give it to the wives and children and the dependants. For extreme need, the older Poor Law still exists. For some particular groups there are other facilities. But for something like half the population, the first-line health service of a personal medical adviser depends on what private arrangements any particular person can manage to make.

Even if a person has a regular doctor – and this is not now assured to all – there is no guaranteed link between that doctor and the rest of necessary medical help. The doctor, both in private practice and in National Health Insurance practice, has to rely on his own resources to introduce his patient to the right kinds of special treatment or clinic or hospital – a great responsibility in these days of specialised medicine and surgery – or the patient has to make his own way to whatever local authority or other organisation happens to cater for his particular need.

When a hospital's services are needed, it is far from true that everyone can get all that is required. Here it is not so much a question of people not being eligible to get the service which they need, as a matter of the practical distribution of those services. The hospital and specialist services have grown up without a national or even an area plan. In one area there may be already established a variety of hospitals. Another area, although the need is there, may be sparsely served. One hospital may have a long waiting list and be refusing admission to cases which another hospital not far away could suitably accommodate and treat at once. There is undue pressure in some areas on the hospital out-patient departments – in spite of certain experiments which some of the hospitals have tried (and which should be encouraged) in arranging a system of timed appointments to obviate long waiting. Moreover, even though most people have access to a hospital of some kind, it is not necessarily access to the right hospital. The tendency in the modern development of medicine and surgery is towards specialist centres – for radiotherapy and neurosis, for example – and no one hospital can be equally equipped and developed to suit all needs, or to specialise equally in all subjects. The time has come when the hospital services have to be thought of, and planned, as a wider whole, and the object has to be that each case should be referred not to one single hospital which happens to be 'local' but to whatever hospital concentrates specially on that kind of case and can offer it the most up-to-date technique.

Many services are also rendered by local authorities and others in special clinics and similar organisations, designed for particular groups of the population or for particular kinds of ailment or medical care. These are, for the most part, thoroughly good in themselves, and they are used with advantage by a great many people in a great many districts. But, owing to the way in which they have grown up piecemeal at different stages of history and under different statutory powers, they are usually conducted as quite separate and independent services. There is no sufficient link either between these services themselves or between them and general medical practice and the hospitals.

In short, general medical practice, consultant and specialist opinion, hospital treatment, clinic services for particular purposes, home nursing, midwifery and other branches of health care need to be related to one another and treated as many aspects of the care of one person's health. That means that there has to be somewhere a new responsibility to relate them, if a service for health is to be given in future which will be not only comprehensive and reliable but also easy to obtain.

Last, but not least, personal health still tends to be regarded as something to be treated when at fault, or perhaps to be preserved from getting at fault, but seldom as something to be positively improved and promoted and made full and robust. Much of present custom and habit still centres on the idea that the doctor and the hospital and the clinic are the means of mending ill-health rather than of increasing good health and the sense of well-being. While the health standards of the people have enormously improved, and while there are the gratifying reductions in the ravages of preventable disease, the plain fact remains that there are many men and women and children who could be and ought to be enjoying a sense of health and physical well-being which they do not in fact enjoy. There is much subnormal health still, which need not be, with a corresponding cost in efficiency and personal happiness.

These are some of the chief deficiencies in the present arrangements which, in the view of the Government, a comprehensive health service should seek to make good . . .

The Scope of a 'Comprehensive' Service

The proposed service must be 'comprehensive' in two senses – first, that it is available to all people and, second, that it covers all necessary forms of health care. The general aim has been stated at the beginning of this Paper. The service designed to achieve it must cover the whole field of medical advice and attention, at home, in the consulting room, in the hospital or the sanatorium, or wherever else is appropriate – from the personal or family doctor to the specialists and consultants of all kinds, from the care of minor ailments to the care of major diseases and disabilities. It must include ancillary services of nursing, of midwifery and of the other things which ought to go with medical care. It must secure first that everyone can be sure of a general medical adviser to consult as and when the need arises, and then that everyone can get access – beyond the general medical adviser – to more specialised branches of medicines or surgery. This cannot all be perfected at a stroke of the pen, on an appointed day; but nothing less than this must be the object in view, and the framing of the service from the outset must be such as to make it possible.

From: Ministry of Health (1944), *A National Health Service*, Cmd 6502, London: HMSO, pp. 6–9, reproduced by permission.

Appendix Three

Aneurin Bevan (Labour) and Richard Law (Conservative) debate the introduction of the National Health Service

Mr Bevan: The first reason why a health scheme of this sort is necessary to all is because it has been the firm conclusion of all parties that money ought not to be permitted to stand in the way of obtaining an efficient health service. Although it is true that the national health insurance system provides a general practitioner service and caters for something like 21 million of the population, the rest of the population have to pay whenever they desire the services of a doctor. It is cardinal to a proper health organisation that a person ought not to be financially deterred from seeking medical assistance at the earliest possible stage. It is one of the evils of having to buy medical advice that in addition to the natural anxiety that may arise because people do not like to hear unpleasant things about themselves, and therefore tend to postpone consultation as long as possible, there is the financial anxiety caused by having to pay doctors' bills. Therefore, the first evil that we must deal with is that which exists as a consequence of the fact that the whole thing is the wrong way round. A person ought to be able to receive medical and hospital help without being involved in financial anxiety.

In the second place, the national health insurance scheme does not provide for the self-employed, nor, of course, for the families of dependants. It depends on insurance qualification, and no matter how ill you are; if you cease to be insured you cease to have free doctoring. Furthermore, it gives no backing to the doctor in the form of specialist services. The doctor has to provide himself, he has to use his own discretion and his own personal connections, in order to obtain hospital treatment for his patient and in order to get them specialists, and in very many cases, of course – in an overwhelming number of cases – the services of a specialist are not available to poor people.

Not only is this the case, but our hospital organisation has grown up with no plan, with no system; it is unevenly distributed over the country and indeed it is one of the tragedies of the situation, that very often the best hospital facilities are available where they are least needed. In the older industrial districts of Great Britain hospital facilities are inadequate. Many of the hospitals are too small – very much too small.

Furthermore – I want to be quite frank with the House – I believe it is repugnant to a civilised community for hospitals to have to rely upon private charity. I believe we ought to have left hospital flag days behind. I have always felt a shudder of repulsion when I have seen nurses and sisters who ought to be at their work, and students who ought to be at their work, going about the streets collecting money for the hospitals. I do not believe there is an Honourable Member of this House who approves that system. It is repugnant, and we must leave it behind – entirely. But the implications of doing this are very considerable.

I have been forming some estimates of what might happen to voluntary hospital finance when the all-in insurance contributions fail to be paid by the people of Great Britain, when the Bill is passed and becomes an Act and they are entitled to free hospital services. The estimates I have go to show that between 80% and 90% of the revenues of the voluntary hospitals in these circumstances will be provided by public funds, by national or rate funds. (An Hon. Member: 'By workers' contributions'). And, of course, as the Honourable Member reminds me, in the very many parts of the country it is a travesty to call them voluntary hospitals. In the mining districts, in the textile districts, in the districts where there are heavy industries it is the industrial population who pay the weekly contributions for the maintenance of the hospitals. When I was a miner I used to find that situation, when I was on the hospital committee. We had an annual meeting and a cordial vote of thanks was moved and passed with great enthusiasm to the managing director of the colliery company for his generosity towards the hospital; and when I looked at the balance sheet, I saw that 97.5% of the revenues were provided by the miners' own contributions; but nobody passed a vote of thanks to the miners . . .

Mr Law: . . . We accept the principle, and we accept the consequences that flow from it. We understand, for example, that once we are committed, as we are gladly committed, to the principle of a 100% service, we require an enormous expansion and development in the health services as a whole. We understand, once we accept the principle, that we are committed to a far greater degree of coordination, or planning as it is usually called, than we have ever known before . . . if my Right Honourable and learned friend the Member for North Croydon (Mr Willink) had still been Minister of Health, had the General Election result gone another way, I do not doubt that he would have introduced, before this, a Bill which would have differed from this Bill only in that my Right Honourable and learned friend would not have attempted to control, own and direct the hospital services of this country or to interfere with that age-old relationship which exists, always has existed, and in our view ought to continue to exist, between a doctor and his patient. Therefore, the Right Honourable Gentleman is not entitled to say – he has not said it, but he might – that we will the end without the means. We will both the end and the means. We will this end, a comprehensive and efficient health service. We are willing to support any practicable means that will give us that end.

But we differ from the Right Honourable Gentleman on this issue. We believe that the Right Honourable Gentleman could have reached his end, and a better end, by other means, and by better means. We believe that he could have established a health service, equally comprehensive, better coordinated and far more efficient, if he had not been determined to sweep away the voluntary hospitals; if he had not been determined to weaken the whole structure of English local government by removing from the field of local government one of the most important and vital responsibilities of local authorities; and if he had not sought to impose upon the medical profession a form of discipline which, in our view and in theirs, is totally unsuited to the practice of medicine, an art, a vocation, however you like to call it, which depends above all else upon individual responsibility, individual devotion and individual sympathy.

From: *Hansard*, 30 April 1946, with permission.

Appendix Four

National Health Service Bill, 1946

Introductory

1. The Bill provides for the establishment of a comprehensive health service in England and Wales. A further Bill to provide for Scotland will be introduced later.
2. The Bill does not deal in detail with everything involved in the service. It deals with the main structure. Within that structure, further provision will be made by statutory regulations – on lines which the Bill lays down and subject always to the control of Parliament.

Scope of the service

3. The Bill provides for the following kinds of health services:
    i) Hospital and specialist services – i.e. all forms of general and special hospital provision, including mental hospitals, together with sanatoria, maternity accommodation, treatment during convalescence, medical rehabilitation and other institutional treatment. These cover in-patient and out-patient services, the latter including clinics and dispensaries operated as part of any specialist service. The advice and services of specialists of all kinds are also to be made available, where necessary, at health centres and in the patient's home.
    ii) Health Centres and general practitioner services – i.e. general personal health care by doctors and dentists whom the patient chooses. These personal practitioner services are to be available both from new publicly equipped health centres and also from the practitioners' own surgeries.
    iii) Various supplementary services – including midwifery, maternity and child welfare, health visiting, home-nursing, a priority dental service for children and expectant and nursing mothers, domestic help where needed on health grounds, vaccination and immunisation against infectious diseases, additional special care and after-care in cases of illness, ambulance services, blood transfusion and laboratory services. (Special school health services are already provided for in the Education Act of 1944).
    iv) The provision of spectacles, dentures and other appliances, together with drugs and medicines – at hospitals, health centres, clinics, pharmacists' shops and elsewhere, as may be appropriate.

Availability of the service

4. All the service, or any part of it, is to be available to everyone in England and Wales. The Bill imposes no limitations on availability – e.g. limitations based on financial means, age, sex, employment or vocation, areas of residence, or insurance qualification.
5. The last is important. If the National Insurance Bill now before Parliament is passed into law, almost everyone will become compulsorily insurable, and after payment of the appropriate contributions will become entitled to the various cash benefits – including sickness and maternity benefits – for which that Bill provides. A proportion of their contributions will be used to help to finance the health services under the present Bill, but the various health service benefits under the present Bill are not made conditional upon any insurance qualification or the proof of having paid contributions. There are no waiting or qualifying periods.
6. The service is to be available from a date to be declared by Order in Council under the Bill, and it is hoped that this will be at the beginning of the year 1948.

The service to be free of fees or charges

7. The health service is to be financed partly from the exchequer, partly from local rates, partly from the help (mentioned above) which part of the National Insurance contributions will give. There are to be no fees or charges to the patient, with the following exceptions:
    i) There will be some charges (to be prescribed later by regulations) for the renewal or repair of spectacles, dentures and other appliances, where this is made necessary through negligence in the care of the articles provided.
    ii) There will be charges (taking into account ability to pay) for the provision of domestic help under the Bill and for certain goods or articles (e.g. supplementary foods, blankets, etc) which may be provided in connection with maternity and child welfare or the special care or after-care of the sick.
    iii) It will be open to people if they wish, in certain cases, to pay for additional amenities within the arrangements of the service – e.g. to pay extra for articles or appliances of higher cost than those normally made available, or to pay charges for private rooms in hospitals (which they will nevertheless be able to obtain free where privacy is medically necessary).

General organisation of the service

8. The Bill places a general duty upon the Minister of Health to promote a comprehensive health service for the improvement of the physical and

mental health of the people of England and Wales, and for the prevention, diagnosis and treatment of illness. To bring physical and mental health closer together in a single service, it transfers to the Minister the present administrative functions of the Board of Control in regard to mental health (the Board retaining only its quasi-judicial functions connected with the liberty of the subject).

From: *The National Health Service Bill* (1946), Cmd 6761, London: HMSO, reproduced by permission.

Appendix Five

Objectives of the NHS in 1979

The Merrison Commission outlined the objectives of the NHS in the following way:

Encouraging and Assisting Individuals to Remain Healthy

We consider it legitimate and positively desirable to devote public resources to the maintenance and promotion of personal as well as public health, not only by the constraints of law but also by offering exhortation, education and incentives. The NHS cannot cover the whole field. Though protracted unemployment and poor social conditions may impair the quality of life and health, it is the responsibility of the organs of government to promote employment and to care for the environment. The encouragement and advancement of good personal health is vitally important . . . It is a proper objective of the NHS to keep the individual in good health.

Equality of Entitlement

We consider, like the framers of the original legislation, that the NHS should be available without restriction by age, social class, sex, race or religion to all people living in the UK.* We are in no doubt that one of the most significant achievements of the NHS has been to free people from fear of being unable to afford treatment for acute or chronic illness, but we regret that they must often wait too long for such treatment.

A Broad Range of Services of High Standard

This is perhaps the most difficult matter we have to discuss and it is at the heart of our terms of reference. We deal with it more fully in Part II of the report, but our definition of this objective includes health promotion, disease prevention, cure, care and after care. The NHS was, from the first, designed to be a comprehensive service. The 1944 White Paper said:

---

* We propose no change in policy towards providing treatment to non-residents of the UK. It is right that those who fall ill while they are in this country should continue to receive treatment under the NHS but that unless there is a reciprocal agreement with a particular country a charge should be made if treatment is specifically sought in the UK.

> The proposed service must be 'comprehensive' in two senses – first, that it is available to all people and, second, that it covers all necessary forms of health care.

The impossibility of meeting all demands for health services was not anticipated. Medical, nursing and therapeutic techniques have been developed to levels of sophistication and expense which were not foreseen when the NHS was introduced.

Standards of cure and care within a given level of resources are in practice largely in the hands of the health professions. They are nevertheless of the greatest concern to the patient. The aim must always be to raise standards in areas where there are deficiencies, but not at the expense of places where services are already good. The NHS has achieved much. It should remain an objective of a national health service to see that it has an active role in disseminating high standards. Sir George Godber, Chief Medical Officer at the Department of Health and Social Security 1960–73, puts the point thus:

> The burden upon the NHS is that of generalization from the example of the best and the result of having such a national service should be the more rapid development of improved services available to all.

Equality of Access

It is unrealistic to suppose that people in all parts of the United Kingdom can have equal ease of access to all services of an identical standard. Access to the highest standard of care will be limited by the numbers of those who can provide such care. There are parts of the country which are better or worse provided with services than others. We draw attention . . . to the special problems of rural areas and declining urban areas . . . Nonetheless, a fundamental purpose of a national service must be equality of provision so far as this can be achieved without an unacceptable sacrifice of standards . . .

A Service Free at the Time of Use

Charges for services within the NHS have always been a matter of controversy, and have led on occasion to the resignation of ministers . . . there are three points to be made here. First, the purpose of charges may be to raise revenue, or discourage the frivolous use of the service, or both. Second, charges may be made for a service which, though provided by or through the NHS, is not essential to the care or treatment of patients – for example, amenity beds in NHS hospitals. Third, in any consideration of charges, it is important to stress that 'free at the time of use' is quite different from 'free'. We do not have a free health service; we have a service to which all taxpayers, employees and employers contribute, regardless of the use they make of it. The effect of this is that those members of the community who do not require extensive use of the NHS help to pay for the care of those who do. It is worth remembering that about 60% of the total expenditure of the NHS goes on children, the old, the disabled, the mentally ill and the mentally handicapped.

Satisfying Reasonable Expectations

This objective can be considered from the point of view of the individual patient, or more generally. Most patients lack the technical knowledge to make informed judgements about diagnosis and treatment. Ignorance may as easily be a reason for a patient being satisfied with his treatment as for his being dissatisfied. One aspect of care on which he will be reliable, however, is whether he has been humanely treated. While doctors are properly deferred to as experts on the technical aspects of medicine, options, when they exist, should be carefully explained and wherever feasible the choice of treatment left to the patient and his relatives. Maximum freedom of choice seems to us an important aspect of this objective although we recognise that there may sometimes be practical limitations on complete freedom of choice for patients. A patient, or potential patient, who is capable of deciding for himself, should be free to:

- consult a doctor, dentist, or other health professional;
- change his practitioner;
- choose a particular hospital or unit with the help of his general practitioner, and
- refuse treatment or advice where the health or safety of others would be endangered.

More generally, it is important for any health service to carry its users with it, given that it can never satisfy all the demands made upon it. It is misleading to pretend that the NHS can meet all expectations. Hard choices have to be made. It is a prime duty of those concerned in the provision of health care to make it clear to the rest of us what we can reasonably expect.

A National Service Responsive to Local Needs

Health services meet different situations in different parts of the country. The range, speed of development and pattern of service delivery will need to vary. Some services can best be provided on a national or regional basis; specialised treatment may require complicated equipment and a higher degree of expertise than can be provided in every community. But if inflexibility is to be avoided, health authorities should implement national policy in the context of their particular geographical and demographic constraints.

From: Merrison, A. (Chairman) (1979) *Report of the Royal Commission on the National Health Service*, Cmnd 7615, London: HMSO, pp. 9–12, reproduced by permission.

Appendix Six

Keith Joseph's Rationale for Proposed Reorganisation in 1974 National Health Service Reorganisation: England

Foreword

For two years I have been responsible for the National Health Service – and for the personal social services.

Throughout this time my respect for the achievements of the National Health Service has steadily grown. Whatever its defects we would be utterly wrong to take for granted the massive performance of this remarkable network of services and the ease of mind that it has brought to all the people of this country. I am sure that they feel a deep sense of gratitude to all those involved: to the members of the governing authorities; to the men and women who make their careers in the service, whether in direct contact with patients or in supporting services; and to the voluntary workers.

But at the same time I have come to recognise, as many others have, that while this good work will continue, nothing like its full potential can be realised without changes in the administrative organisation of the service.

Hence this White Paper. It is about administration, not about treatment and care. But the purpose behind the changes proposed is a better, more sensitive, service to the public. Administration is not of course an end in itself. But both the patients and those who provide treatment and care will gain if the administration embodies both a clear duty to improve the service and the facilities for doing so.

Let me illustrate this. Everyone is aware of gaps in our health services. Even for acute illness, where we provide at least as good a service for our whole population as any country in the world, there are some respects in which we achieve less than we could. On the non-acute side the service for the elderly, for the disabled, and for the mentally ill and the mentally handicapped have failed to attract the attention and indeed the resources which they need – and all the more credit to the staff who have toiled so tirelessly for their patients despite the difficulties.

It is well understood now, moreover, that the domiciliary and community services are under-developed – that there is a need for far more home helps, home nurses, hostels and day centres and other services that support people outside hospital. Often what there is could achieve more if it were better co-ordinated with other services in and out of hospital. It is well understood too that there must be more emphasis on prevention – or at the least on early detection and treatment.

For the imbalances and the gaps Governments must take their share of the responsibility. Resources were and still are stretched. The acute services had a legitimate priority. But the shortcomings were not rational. They did not result from a calculation as to the best way to deploy scarce resources. They just happened.

Why did they just happen? Because it has never been the responsibility – nor has it been within the power – of any single named authority to provide for the population of a given area of a comprehensible size the best health service that the money and skills available can provide. There has been no identified authority whose task it has been, in co-operation with those responsible for complementary services, to balance needs and priorities nationally and to plan and provide the right combination of services for the benefit of the public.

It is to enable such an authority to operate in each area, with the best professional advice, that the Government proposes to reorganise the administration of the National Health Service as explained in this White Paper.

The National Health Service is one of the largest civilian organisations in the world. Its staff is growing rapidly. It contains an ever-growing multitude of skills that depend on and interact with each other. It serves an ever-growing range of health needs with ever more complex treatments and techniques.

And though the Government has made substantial additions to a programme of expenditure which has already planned to grow at an above-average rate, there is never enough money – and never likely to be – for everything that ideally requires to be done. Nor, despite the great increase since 1948, are there ever enough skilled men and women.

Real needs must therefore be identified, and decisions must be taken and periodically reviewed, as to the order of priorities among them. Plans must be worked out to meet these needs and management and drive must be continually applied to put the plans into action, assess their effectiveness and modify them as needs change or as ways are found to make the plans more effective.

Effective for what? – to improve the service for the benefit of all. The plans must therefore be effective in providing what patients need: primarily, treatment and care in hospital; support at home; diagnosis and treatment in surgery, health centre or out-patient clinic; or day care.

Furthermore they must include arrangements whereby the public can express their wishes and preferences, and know that notice will be taken of them. That is why I attach great importance to the establishment of strong community health councils, and to improved methods for enquiring into complaints, including the appointment of a health ombudsman.

The health services depend crucially on the humane planning and provision of the personal social services, and therefore on effective and understanding collaboration with local government. No doubt arguments will continue about the theoretical advantages of making both health and social services the responsibility of a single agency. But the formidable practical difficulties, which have been fully argued elsewhere, rule this out as a realistic solution, and require us to concentrate instead on ensuring that the two parallel authorities – one local, one health – with their separate statutory responsibilities shall work together in partnership for the health and social care of the population. This

White Paper demonstrates the Government's concern to see that arrangements are evolved under which a more coherent and smoothly interlocking range of services will develop for all the needs of the population.

The doctor and other professional workers will gain too. The organisational changes will not affect the professional relationship between individual patients and individual professional workers on which the complex of health services is so largely built. The professional workers will retain their clinical freedom – governed as it is by the bounds of professional knowledge and ethics and by the resources that are available – to do as they think best for their patients. This freedom is cherished by the professions and accepted by the Government. It is a safeguard for patients today and an insurance for future improvements.

But the organisational changes will also bring positive gains to the professional worker. He – or she – will have the opportunity of organising his or her own work better and of playing a much greater part than hitherto in the management decisions that are taken in each area. At the same time the more systematic and comprehensive analysis of needs and priorities that will lie behind the planning and operations of each area will help professional workers to ensure their skills bring the greatest possible benefit to their patients.

We are issuing a White Paper and promoting legislation about the administration of the National Health Service, solely in order to improve the health care of the public. Administrative reorganisation within a unified health service that is closely linked with parallel local government services will provide a sure foundation for better services for all.

Keith Joseph
Secretary of State for Social Services

From: *National Health Service Reorganisation: England* (1972), Cmnd 5055, London: HMSO, pp. v–vii, reproduced by permission.

Appendix Seven

The 2nd RAWP Report Outlining the Basis for Allocating Resources

Introduction and Background

1.1 There is ample evidence to demonstrate that demand for health care throughout the world is rising inexorably. England has no immunity from this phenomenon. And because it can also be shown that supply of health care actually fuels further demand, it is inevitable that the supply of health care services can never keep pace with the rising demands placed upon them. Demand will always be one jump ahead. This is a problem for Government and society in general and not, fortunately, one to which the Working Party was called upon to address its mind. We mention it at the beginning of this Report, however, to emphasize two points. Firstly that the resources available to the NHS are bound to fall short of requirements as measured by demand criteria and secondly that supply of facilities has an important influence on demand in the locality in which they are provided.

1.2 Supply of health facilities is, in England as elsewhere, also variable and very much influenced by history. The methods used to distribute financial resources to the NHS have, since its inception, tended to reflect the inertia built into the system by history. They have tended to increment the historic basis for the supply of real resources (e.g. facilities and manpower); and, by responding comparatively slowly and marginally to changes in demography and morbidity, have also tended to perpetuate the historic situation.

1.3 This led us in our Interim Report to interpret the underlying objective of our terms of reference as being to secure, through resource allocation, that there would eventually be equal opportunity of access to health care for people at equal risk. We reaffirm this view. It has involved us in seeking criteria which are broadly responsive to relative need, not supply or demand, and to employ those criteria to establish and quantify in a relative way the differentials of need between different geographical locations. For practical purposes these geographic locations must correspond with those into which the NHS is organized to administer the delivery of health care, viz, Regions, Areas and Districts.

1.4 In searching for criteria which are responsive in this way, we have had perforce to consider only those criteria, the supporting statistical data for which are readily available and reliable at all three levels of disaggregation required. We have further taken as an aim the desirability of keeping the methods proposed as simple as possible, consistent with the overall objective. The degree of refinement necessary is to some extent a matter of judgement, but we have not by any means regarded perfection in this context as an aim. On the contrary, we have rejected many approaches which might have made the criteria more sensitive, but which on examination would have led to much greater complexity with little significant change in the result.

1.5   **Resource allocation is concerned with the distribution of financial resources which are used for the provision of real resources. In this sense it is concerned with the means rather than the end. We have not regarded our remit as being concerned with how the resources are deployed.** This must be a matter for the administering Authorities and is essentially part of their policy-making, planning and decision-making functions in response to central guidelines on national policies and priorities. Resource allocation will clearly have an important influence on the discharge of those functions and be the most critical guideline within which they have to be discharged. This serves, however, to emphasize the importance, as our terms of reference direct, of ensuring that the availability of the finite resource at the NHS's disposal should be determined in relation to criteria of need.

Criteria of Need

Size of Population

1.6   Health care is for people and clearly the primary determinant of need must be the size of the population. This must therefore be the basic divisor used to distribute the resource available to each level required.

Population Make-up

1.7   The make-up of the population is, however, critical. People do not have identical needs for health care. For example, the elderly (men and women aged 65 and over) form about 14% of the total population, yet they occupy more than half the non-psychiatric hospital beds (excluding maternity). Women have needs different to men, and children too are heavy users of health care facilities. Similarly, patterns of morbidity are different between the sexes at different ages. Thus the age/sex make-up of the population needs to be taken into account as well as its size.

Morbidity

1.8   Even when differences due to age and sex are fully accounted for, populations of the same size and make-up display different morbidity characteristics. The reasons are simple enough to guess but harder to quantify; environment, social circumstances, heredity, occupation etc. all play a part. But a population-based measure of need which takes no account of different patterns of morbidity would ignore geographic variations which, on the data available, are significant.

Cost

1.9 The costs of providing care in response to need are also variable. Some conditions are very expensive to treat, others less so. It is not enough to use criteria which predict the likely incidence of the more expensive forms of care, unless at the same time some account is taken of the differential cost involved. Furthermore, the costs of exactly the same form of care may vary from place to place depending on local variations in market forces. A clear example of this is the weighting paid to staff employed in the London area.

Health Care Across Administrative Boundaries

1.10 The populations for which the administering Authorities are responsible for delivering health care are primarily those who reside within their geographic boundaries. In some cases these responsibilities are adjusted to take account of people residing in overlap areas – by means of formal agency or extra-territorial management arrangements. For resource allocation purposes the population needs to be that for which the Authority exercises a management responsibility.

1.11 But these arrangements do not take account of patients who receive care outside the managed area of their particular Authority. Patient flows across boundaries result from the fact that few Areas and Districts are entirely self-sufficient in terms of the services they provide. In some cases these 'deficiencies' are planned, e.g. regional specialties, in others they are unplanned and are often the inevitable consequence of new and arbitrary administrative boundaries not matching established patterns of health care delivery. To a large extent unplanned patient flows are also a measure of geographical disparity in health care provision. Whether patient flows are from choice or necessity, the populations used for revenue allocations need to be adjusted to take account of the movement. And such adjustment ought also to reflect the different costs of care involved.

Medical and Dental Education

1.12 The NHS has a responsibility to provide clinical facilities for the teaching of students qualifying through the University Medical Schools. Service facilities which are used for medical and dental education are more costly to provide. The incidence of these costs is, however, unrelated either to the size or to the needs of the populations served by the hospitals where medical and dental education is undertaken. Means must therefore be found of identifying the additional costs necessarily involved and protecting those costs from the effects of allocation processes based upon population and service need criteria.

Capital Investment

1.13 Health services require considerable capital investment in buildings, plant and equipment. Whilst the need for capital investment may to a considerable extent be measurable by criteria similar to those used for determining need for current expenditure, there is one significant difference. As mentioned earlier in this chapter, the distribution of capital stock is still very much influenced by the historic patterns of health care delivery. There are not only geographic inequalities in the quantity of stock available but also in its age and condition. Nor do these factors of quantity and quality go hand in hand. Regions which are well provided in quantitative terms may, for the same historic reasons, have a large proportion of ageing stock. Furthermore, the effects of population movement, demographic change and the redefinition of administrative boundaries have all exacerbated the 'mislocation' problem.

From: DHSS (1976) *Sharing Resources for Health in England,* Report of the Resource Allocation Working Party, London: HMSO, pp. 7–10, reproduced by permission.

Reference

Allsop, J. (1984) *Health Policy and the National Health Service,* London and New York: Longman.

Appendix Eight

Working for Patients

Foreword by the Prime Minister

The National Health Service at its best is without equal. Time and again, the nation has seen just how much we owe to those who work in it.

A skilled and dedicated staff – backed by enormously increased resources – have coped superbly with the growing demands of modern medicine and increasing numbers of patients. There is a great deal of which we can all feel very proud.

The National Health Service will continue to be available to all, regardless of income, and to be financed mainly out of general taxation.

But major tasks now face us: to bring all parts of the National Health Service up to the very high standard of the best, while maintaining the principles on which it was founded; and to prepare for the needs of the future.

We aim to extend patient choice, to delegate responsibility to where the services are provided and to secure the best value for money.

All proposals in this White Paper put the needs of patients first.

They apply to the whole of the United Kingdom but there are separate chapters on Scotland, Wales and Northern Ireland to cater for their special circumstances.

We believe that a National Health Service that is run better, will be a National Health Service that can care better.

Taken together, the proposals represent the most far-reaching reform of the National Health Service in its 40-year history.

They offer new opportunities, and pose new challenges, for everyone concerned with the running of the service.

I am confident that all who work in it will grasp these opportunities to provide even **better** health care for the millions and millions of people who rely on the National Health Service.

The patient's needs will always be paramount.

Margaret Thatcher

The Need for Change

1.4   Throughout the 1980s the Government has thus presided over a massive expansion of the NHS. It has ensured that the quality of care provided and the response to emergencies remain among the best in the world. But it has become increasingly clear that more needs to be done because of rising demand and an ever-widening range of treatments made possible by advances in medical technology. It has also increasingly been recognised that simply injecting more and more money is not, by itself, the answer.

1.5   It is clear that the organisation of the NHS – the way it delivers health care to the individual patient – also needs to be reformed. The Government has been tackling these organisational problems, and has taken a series of measures to improve the way the NHS is managed. The main one was the introduction of general management from 1984. This is now showing results and has pointed the way ahead.

1.6   New management information systems have provided clear evidence of a wide variation in performance up and down the country. In 1986–87, the average cost of treating acute hospital in-patients varied by as much as 50% between different health authorities, even after allowing for the complexity and mix of cases treated. Similarly, a patient who waits several years for an operation in one place may get that same operation within a few weeks in another. There are wide variations in the drug prescribing habits of GPs, and in some places drug costs are nearly twice as high per head of population as in others. And, at the extremes, there is a 20-fold variation in the rate at which GPs refer patients to hospital.

The Government's Proposals

Key Changes

1.9   The Government is proposing seven key measures to achieve these objectives:

First: **to make the Health Service more responsive to the needs of patients, as much power and responsibility as possible will be delegated to local level.** This includes the delegation of functions from Regions to Districts, and from Districts to hospitals. The detailed proposals are set out in the next chapter. They include greater flexibility in setting the pay and conditions of staff, and financial incentives to make the best use of a hospital's assets.

Second: **to stimulate a better service to the patient, hospitals will be able to apply for a new self-governing status as NHS Hospital Trusts.** This means that, while remaining within the NHS, they will take fuller responsibility for their own affairs, harnessing the skills and dedication of their staff. NHS Hospital Trusts will earn revenue from the services they provide. They will therefore have an incentive to attract patients, so they will make sure that the service they offer is what their patients want. And in turn they will stimulate other NHS hospitals to respond to what people want locally. NHS Hospital Trusts will also be able to set the rates of pay of their own staff and, within annual financing limits, to borrow money to help them respond to patient demand.

Third: **to enable hospitals which best meet the needs and wishes of patients to get the money to do so, the money required to treat patients will be able to cross administrative boundaries.** All NHS hospitals, whether run by health authorities or self-governing, will be free to offer their services to different health authorities and to the private sector. Consequently, a health authority will be better able to discharge its duty to use its available funds to secure a comprehensive service, including emergency services, by obtaining the best service it can whether from its own hospitals, from another authority's hospitals, from NHS Hospital Trusts or from the private sector.

Sixth: **to improve the effectiveness of NHS management, regional, district and family practitioner management bodies will be reduced in size and reformed on business lines, with executive and non-executive directors.** The Government believes that, in the interests of patients and staff, the era in which a £26 billion NHS is run by authorities which are neither truly representative nor fully management bodies must be ended. The confusion of roles will be replaced by a clear remit and accountability.

Seventh: **to ensure that all concerned with delivering services to the patient make the best use of the resources available to them, quality of service and value for money will be more rigorously audited.** Arrangements for what doctors call 'medical audit' will be extended throughout the Health Service, helping to ensure that the best quality of medical care is given to patients. The Audit Commission will assume responsibility for auditing the accounts of health authorities and other NHS bodies, and will undertake wide-ranging value for money studies.

The Best Use of Resources

1.15 If the NHS is to provide the best service it can for its patients, it must make the best use of the resources available to it. The quest for value for money must be an essential element in its work. This becomes even more important as the demands on the Health Service continue to grow.

1.16 Those who take decisions which involve spending money must be accountable for that spending. Equally, those who are responsible for managing the service must be able to influence the way in which its resources are used. The Government believes that most decisions are better taken at local level.

From: *Working for Patients* (1989), CM 555, London: HMSO, pp. Foreword–8, reproduced by permission.

References and Footnotes

1. Allsop, J. (1984) *Health Policy and the National Health Service*, London and New York: Longman.
2. Seedhouse, D. F. (1991) A Right to be Heard: An Interview with Graham Pink, *Health Matters*, 8: 25.
3. HMSO (1992) Guidelines on Freedom of Speech for NHS Staff, Summary, *Bulletin of Medical Ethics*, 83: 9–11.
4. Twycross, R. G. (1980) Hospice Care – Redressing the Balance in Medicine, *Journal of the Royal Society of Medicine*, 73: 475–481.
5. Strong, P. and Robinson, J. (1990) *The NHS: Under New Management*, Milton Keynes, Open University Press.
6. Maynard, A. and Hutton, J. (1992) Health Care Reform: The Search for the Holy Grail, *Health Economics*, 1: 1–3.
7. Cribb, A. (1993) The Borders of Health Promotion, *Health Care Analysis*, 1(2), 131–137.
8. Seedhouse, D. F. (1991) *Liberating Medicine*, Chichester: John Wiley & Sons.
9. Nordenfelt, L. (1993) On the nature and ethics of health promotion. An attempt at systematic analysis, *Health Care Analysis*, 1,(2), 121–130.
10. Moore, A., Hope, T. and Fulford, K. W. M. (1993) Mild Mania and Well-Being, *Philosophy, Psychiatry and Psychology*, (forthcoming).
11. Palmer, R. L. (1988) *Anorexia Nervosa: A Guide for Sufferers and their Families*, Harmondsworth: Penguin.
12. Kleidan, O. (1963) The Health Services, in A. Forder (ed.) *Penelope Hall's Social Services of England and Wales*, p. 137.
13. Parker, J. (1965) *Local Health and Welfare Services*, London: Allen and Unwin, p. 70.
14. Aneurin Bevan quoted in *Hansard*, 20 April 1946.
15. Ministry of Health (1920) *Interim Report on the Future Provision of Medical and Allied Services*, Cmd 693, London: HMSO.
16. Klein, R. (1989) *The Politics of the National Health Service*, 2nd edition, London and New York: Longman, pp. 10–11.
17. Ministry of Health (1944), *A National Health Service*, Cmd 6502, London: HMSO.
18. Public Records Office, MH 80/24, Minutes of the first of a series of office conferences on the development of health services, dated 7 February 1938; Minutes by the Chief Medical Officer, dated 21 September 1939.
19. Klein, R. (1989) *The Politics of the National Health Services*, 2nd edition, London and New York: Longman, p. 7.
20. Klein, R. (1989) *The Politics of the National Health Service*, 2nd edition, London and New York: Longman, p. 28.
21. Foucault, M. (1973) *The Birth of the Clinic*. (Translated from the French by A. M. Sheridan Smith), London: Tavistock.
22. NHS Matters (1991) *NHS Support Federation Campaign News*, Issue No. 1.
23. Merrison, A. (Chairman) (1979) *Report of the Royal Commission on the National Health Service*, Cmnd 7615, London: HMSO.

24. *Working for Patients* (1989), 555, London: HMSO.
25. Second Report of the Resource Allocation Working Party – see Appendix Seven.
26. Illiffe, S. (1983) *The NHS: A Picture of Health?*, London: Lawrence and Wishart.
27. Klein, R. (1989) *The Politics of the National Health Service*, 2nd edition, London and New York: Longman, p. 149.
28. Baker, R. (1993) Visibility and the just allocation of health care: A study of dialysis rationing in the British National Health Service, *Health Care Analysis*, 1(2), 139–150.
29. Churchill, R. (1987) *Rationing in Health Care in America: perceptions and principles of justice*, Paris, University of Notre Dame Press. Quoting Aaran, J. and Schwart, W. B. (1984) *The Painful Prescription: Rationing Hospital Care*, Washington D.C.: Brocklyns Institute, pp. 97–99.
30. Hackler, C. (1993) Health Care Reform in the United States, *Health Care Analysis*, 1, 5–13.
31. *Working for Patients. NHS Trusts: A Working Guide* (1984). London: HMSO.
32. NHS Needs-Assessment Job Descriptions, passim.
33. Stevens, A. and Gabbay, J. (1991) Needs Assessment needs assessment, *Health Trends*, 23: 20–23.
34. Liss, P. E. (1990) *Health Care Need. Meaning and Measurement*, Linköping, Sweden: Linköping University, p. 33.
35. Liss, P. E. (1990) *Health Care Need. Meaning and Measurements*, Linköping, Sweden: Linköping University, p. 36.
36. Acheson, D. (1978) The Definition and Identification of Need for Health Care, *Journal of Epidemiology and Community Health*, 32: 10–15.
37. Liss, P. E. (1990) *Health Care Need. Meaning and Measurement*, Linköping, Sweden: Linköping University.
38. Liss, P. E. (1990) *Health Care Need. Meaning and Measurement*, Linköping, Sweden: Linköping University, p. 42.
39. Brazier, M. (1987) *Medicine, Patients and the Law*, Harmondsworth: Penguin.
40. Williams, C. J. (ed.) (1992) *Introducing New Treatments for Cancer: Practical, Ethical and Legal Problems*, Chichester: John Wiley & Sons.
41. Doyal, L. and Gough, I. (1991) *A Theory of Human Need*, London: Macmillan Education Ltd.
42. Thomson, G. (1987) *Needs*, Routledge, Kegan and Paul, London.
43. Liss, P. E. (1990) *Health Care Need. Meaning and Measurement*, Linköping, Sweden: Linköping University, p. 52.
44. Liss, P. E. (1990) *Health Care Need. Meaning and Measurement*, Linköping, Sweden: Linköping University, p. 48.
45. Liss, P. E. (1990) *Health Care Need. Meaning and Measurement*, Linköping, Sweden: Linköping University, p. 81.
46. Thomson, G. (1987) *Needs*, London: Routledge, Kegan and Paul, p. 8.
47. Thomson, G. (1987) *Needs*, London: Routledge, Kegan and Paul, p. 128.
48. Seedhouse, D. F. (1991) *Liberating Medicine*, Chichester: John Wiley & Sons, (see The Category Mistake, pp. 45–50).
49. Seedhouse, D. F. (1991) *Liberating Medicine*, Chichester: John Wiley & Sons, (see Autonomy Flip, pp. 126–129).
50. Brooks, T. (1992) Total Quality Management in the NHS, *Health Services Management*, 18: April 1992.
51. *The Health Services Journal*, passim.
52. See Appendix Eight.
53. Oakland, J. S. (1989) *TQM*, Oxford: Oxford University Press, p. 3.

54. NHS Briefing paper on Quality in the NHS: Source unknown. See also Hill, T., Russell, M., Gill, S., Marchment, M., Morgan, J. and Everett, T. (1990) *Introducing TQM – A Training Manual*, South East Staffs Health Authority.
55. Caplan, R. H. (1988) *A Practical Approach to Quality Control*, 5th edition, London: Random Century Group, p. 4.
56. Deming, W. E. (1986) *Out of the Crisis: Quality, Productivity and Competitive Position*, Cambridge: Cambridge University Press.
57. Juran, J. M. and Gryna, F. M. (1988) *Juran's Quality Control Handbook*, 4th edition, New York: McGraw-Hill.
58. Spencer, B., Morris, J. and Thomas, H. (1989) The South Manchester Family Worker Scheme, in Seedhouse, D. F. and Cribb, A. (eds), *Changing Ideas in Health Care*, Chichester: John Wiley & Sons.
59. Klein, R. (1989) *The Politics of the National Health Service*, 2nd edition, London and New York: Longman, p. 169.
60. Cartwright, F. (1977) *A Social History of Medicine*, London: Longman.
61. Ham, C. (1982) *Health Policy in Britain*, London: Macmillan.
62. See Appendix Seven for example.
63. Lucas, J. R. (1980) *On Justice*, Oxford: Clarendon Press.
64. Norman, R. (1987) *Free and Equal: a Philosophical Examination of Political Values*, Oxford: Oxford University Press.
65. Seedhouse, D. F. (1991) *Liberating Medicine*, Chichester: John Wiley & Sons.
66. Seedhouse, D. F. and Lovett, M. (1992) *Practical Medical Ethics*, Chichester: John Wiley & Sons.
67. Seedhouse, D. F. (1986) *Health: The Foundations for Achievement*, Chichester: John Wiley & Sons.
68. See Appendix One.
69. Seedhouse, D. F. (1991) *Liberating Medicine*, Chichester: John Wiley & Sons, (see the health and disease continua in 'The Category Mistake' section, pp. 126–129).
70. Loewy, E. H. (1980) Cost should not be a factor in medical care, *New England Journal of Medicine*, **302**: 697.
71. Seedhouse, D. F. (1986 and 1991) *Health the Foundations for Achievement* (1986) and *Liberating Medicine* (1991), Chichester: John Wiley & Sons, for a full exposition on this view.
72. Buchanan, I. (1990) Purpose and Process in Health Care: an Examination of Values in the NHS. MSc dissertation in the Ethics of Health Care, University of Liverpool, unpublished.
73. BMA (1987) *Living with Risk*, Chichester: John Wiley & Sons.
74. Spicker, S. F. (1993) Going Off The Dole: A Prudential and Ethical Critique of the Healthfare State, *Health Care Analysis*, **1**, 33–38.
75. Black, D., Townsend, P. and Davidson, N. (1982) *Inequalities in Health: The Black Report*, Harmondsworth: Penguin, p. 29.
76. Ashton, J. (1984) *Health in Mersey – A Review*, Liverpool: University of Liverpool, Department of Community Health (now Public Health).
77. Illiffe, S. (1983) *The NHS: A Picture of Health?*, London: Lawrence and Wishart, see pp. 200–201 for an account of why the Black Report drew back from the obvious, and from some of its expressly stated equalising proposals.
78. Seedhouse, D. F. (1993) Putting the Horse First: the practical value of philosophical analysis, *Health Care Analysis*, **1**, 1–3.
79. Bayer, R., Caplan, A. and Daniels, N. (eds) (1983) *In Search of Equity: Health Needs and the Health Care System*, London: Plenum Press.
80. Tudor Hart, J. (1974) *The NHS in England and Wales*, Communist Party.

81. Tawney, R. H. (1931) *Equality*, London: G. Allen and Unwin Ltd.
82. Harris, J. (1991) Unprincipled QALYs: a response to Cubbon, *Journal of Medical Ethics*, **17**: 185–188.
83. Harris, E. A. (1992) Medical Ethics and the New World Order, *New Zealand Medical Journal*, **105**, 405–407.
84. Sass, H.-M., Massey, R. U. (eds) (1988), *Health Care Systems: Moral Conflicts in European and American Public Policy*, Dordrecht: Kluwer Academic Publishers.
85. Hackler, C. (1993) Health Care Reform in the United States, *Health Care Analysis*, **1**: 5–13; note that the point is arguable.
86. Seedhouse, D. F. (1993) Putting the horse first: the practical value of philosophical analysis, *Health Care Analysis*, **1**, 1–3. (See also HCA passim.)
87. Brannigan, M. (1993) Oregon's Experiment, *Health Care Analysis*, **1**, 15–32.
88. Appendices passim.
89. Griffiths, R. (1992) Seven Years of Progress – General Management in the NHS, *Health Economics*, **1**: 61–70.
90. Appendix Eight.
91. Williams, A. (1992) Cost-Effectiveness Analysis: is it ethical?, *Journal of Medical Ethics*, **18**: 7–11.
92. Culyer, A. (1992) The Morality of Efficiency in Health Care – Some Uncomfortable Implications, *Health Economics*, **1**, 1: 7–18. (See p. 12.)
93. Culyer, A. (1992) The Morality of Efficiency in Health Care – Some Uncomfortable Implications, *Health Economics*, **1**, 1: 7–18. (See p. 8.)
94. Williams, A. (1988) Ethics and Efficiency in the Provision of Health Care, in J. M. Bell and S. Mendus (eds), *Philosophy and Medical Welfare*, Cambridge: Cambridge University Press, p. 112.
95. Maynard, A. and Hutton, J. (1992) Health Care Reform: The Search for the Holy Grail, *Health Economics*, **1**: 1–3. (See the rest of the issue for further evidence.)
96. Boorse, C. (1975) On the distinction between disease and illness, *Philosophy and Public Affairs*, **5**.
97. Nordenfelt, L. (1987) *On the Nature of Health*, Dordrecht: Reidel.
98. Williamson, G., Williams, B., Krekorian, H., McLees, S. and Falloon, I. (1992) QALYs in mental health: a case study, *Psychological Medicine*, **22**: 725–731.
99. Kind, P. K., Rosser, R. M. and Williams, A. (1982) Valuation of Quality of Life: Some Psychometric Evidence', in M. W. Jones-Lee (ed.), *The Value of Life and Safety*, Amsterdam: North Holland Publishing Co.
100. Kind, P. K., Rosser, R. M. and Williams, A. (1982) Valuation of Quality of Life: Some Psychometric Evidence, in M. W. Jones-Lee (ed.), *The Value of Life and Safety*, Amsterdam: North Holland Publishing Co., p. 159.
101. Rosser, R. M. and Kind, P. K. (1978) A Scale of Variations of States of Illness, *International Journal of Epidemiology*, **7**, 4:347–358.
102. Smith, A. (1987) Qualms about QALYs, Department of Epidemiology and Social Oncology, University of Manchester.
103. Gerard. K. and Mooney, G. (1993) QALY League Tables: Handle with Care, *Health Economics*, **2**: 59–64.
104. Williams, A. (1992) Cost-Effectiveness Analysis: is it ethical?, *Journal of Medical Ethics*, **18**: see pages 8–9.
105. Doyal, L. and Pennell, I. (1979) *The Political Economy of Health*, London: Pluto Press.
106. Illich, I. (1977) *Limits to Medicine*, London: Pelican Books.
107. Klein, R. (1989) *The Politics of the National Health Service*, 2nd edition, London and New York: Longman, passim.

108. Navarro, V. 1970) *Medicine Under Capitalism*, London: Croom Helm.
109. Collier, J. (1989) *The Health Conspiracy*, London: Century.
110. Illiffe, S. (1983) *The NHS: A Picture of Health?* London: Lawrence and Wishart, pp. 159–160.
111. Seedhouse, D. F. (1992) The Two Languages of Care, *Journal of Advances in Health and Nursing Care*, **1**, 4: 23–32.
112. Acheson, D. (1978) The Definition and Identification of Need for Health Care, *Journal of Epidemiology and Community Health*, **32**: 10–15. Further representative quotes include: 'If the realistic approach is adopted it would be reasonable and helpful if epidemiologists who set out to measure need for planning purposes could encourage definitions of it to be framed within the constraints determined by service equivalents' and 'To be useful (need) must be defined in terms of the expertise of health professionals and the reasons available at local level to provide such expertise'.
113. *Health Service Journal*, 6 August 1992, p. 12.
114. Towards a General Theory of Health Gain. *Seminar Summary. Proceedings from Health Gain 92: The Standing Conference, Norwich, 23–24 July 1992*.
115. Liddell, A. (1992) Health Gain. *Proceedings from Health Gain 92: The Standing Conference, Norwich, 23–24 July 1992*.
116. See, for example, Institute of Medicine (1990) *Medicare: A Strategy for Quality Assurance*, Vols I and II, Washington: National Academic Press, p. 140.
117. See Appendix Six.
118. Medicaid is a federal and state venture. It is not an entitlement plan since eligibility is not guaranteed. The federal government provides guidelines and contributes a share to each state's funding. However, states administer their programmes as well as set their own eligibility requirements. Eligibility therefore varies among states, and many have set their qualifications quite below the federal poverty level due to constrained state budgets.
119. Callaghan, D. (1987) *Setting Limits: Medical Goals in an Ageing Society*, New York: Touchstone.
120. Menzel, P. (1990) *Strong Medicine: The Ethical Rationing of Health Care*, Oxford: Oxford University Press.
121. Medicare is a federally supported insurance plan for those individuals who are over 65, with permanent disabilities, or with end-stage renal disease. It is an entitlement programme under federal guidelines, and citizens help subsidise it through federal taxes. Certain areas, however, are not covered under Medicare, such as long-term custodial care, prescription drugs, and eye and dental care.
122. Zwart, H. (1993) Rationing in The Netherlands, *Health Care Analysis*, **1**, 53–56.
123. Anon (1993) Individual Responsibility for Health: A Problematic Concept, *Health Promotion International*, (forthcoming).
124. Ashton, T. (1993) From Evolution to Revolution: Restructuring the New Zealand Health System, *Health Care Analysis*, **1**, 57–62.
125. For example, Wennberg, J. (1990) Outcomes Research, Cost Containment, and the Fear of Health Care Rationing, *New England Journal of Medicine*, **323**, 17: 1202–1204.
126. Seedhouse, D. F. (1988) *Ethics: The Heart of Health Care*, Chichester: John Wiley & Sons. (See especially the chapters on 'The Ethical Grid'.)
127. Seedhouse, D. F. (1988) *Ethics: The Heart of Health Care*, Chichester: John Wiley & Sons.
128. Seedhouse, D F. (1991) *Liberating Medicine*, Chichester: John Wiley & Sons. (See 'The Autonomy Flip', pp. 126–129.)

129. Seedhouse, D. F. (1991) *Liberating Medicine*, Chichester: John Wiley & Sons. (See 'The Autonomy Test', Chapter 6.)
130. The AIDS campaign: Every household in England and Wales received a pamphlet describing the dangers of AIDS. This was part of a wider campaign designed, without a doubt, to frighten people into supposedly less 'risky' behaviours.
131. The Poll Tax campaign: In both the AIDS and Poll Tax campaigns, much public money was spent to convince people of the merits of a policy designed by the political party who were in government at the time.
132. Public Charter campaign.
133. The QALY.
134. Beauchamp, T., Childress, L. and James, F. (1983) *Principles of Biomedical Ethics*, 2nd edition, New York: Oxford University Press.
135. *Guardian* leader article, August 1991.
136. Labour Party (1992) *Jennifer's Ear*, Labour Party, Political Broadcast.

Index

Index compiled by Geoffrey C. Jones